Star Quality

The Red Carpet Workout for the Celebrity Body of Your Dreams

ROB PARR

and Laurel House

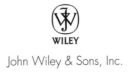

WILEY

John Wiley & Sons, Inc.

Published by John Wiley & Sons, Inc., Hoboken, New Jersey
Published simultaneously in Canada

All photos taken by Jennifer Kennedy of Kennedy Pix.

The information contained in this book is not intended to serve as a replacement for professional medical advice. Any use of the information in this book is at the reader's discretion. The author and the publisher specifically disclaim any and all liability arising directly or indirectly from the use or application of any information contained in this book. A health care professional should be consulted regarding your specific situation.

For general information about our other products and services, please contact our Customer Care Department within the United States at (800) 762-2974, outside the United States at (317) 572-3993 or fax (317) 572-4002.

Wiley also publishes its books in a variety of electronic formats. Some content that appears in print may not be available in electronic books. For more information about Wiley products, visit our web site at www.wiley.com.

ISBN 978-0470-18400-4

Printed in the United States of America

10 9 8 7 6 5 4 3 2 1

To Debra, the wind in my sail and the rudder of my ship

Contents

Acknowledgments

I would like to thank Sharon House, without whose help and guidance this book would not have been possible. Thanks to Stephanie Tade for taking on this project and introducing me to Tom Miller at John Wiley & Sons. Thanks to Laurel House, who took all this information and brought it to life. A very special thanks to all my clients over the past twenty years, who entrusted me with their health and fitness. Thank you, Madonna, Demi Moore, Bruce Willis, John McEnroe, and Naomi Watts for the exposure and opportunities that our relationships have provided to me.

Most important, I thank my wife, Debra, for her support, wisdom, and knowledge of life. She is the wind in my sail and the rudder of my ship, and I'm grateful for all the love she has given me from the beginning of this journey twenty years ago. Our three beautiful children, Jordan, Hunter, and Chandler, have kept me going with all their love and support. Without my family I truly could not continue this type of physical training.

Thank you all for helping me make this book possible.

—Rob Parr

Rob, it was an absolute pleasure—thank you. Mom, your support, strength, encouragement, patience, and therapeutic conversations—both personal and professional—made me who I am and allowed this book to happen. Dad, you introduced me to the world of fitness and taught me to take care of and have pride in my body. Stephanie, thank you for your guidance. Tom Miller, thank you for believing. Gregg, thank you for sharing your knowledge. Thank you, Scott, for your advice and balance. Thank you for your encouragement and love. Thank you for enlivening my spirit.

A special thanks to Sherie Farah, an extremely talented healthy food chef, as well as to our amazing photographer, Jennifer Kennedy with Kennedy Pix. We would also like to thank our gorgeous model, Ambria Miscia with M International, and makeup artist, Monique Hahn.

—Laurel House

Introduction

Are you ready to get in shape? Then get your butt off the couch, slip on and tie up your running shoes, and let's get going!

I'm Rob Parr, and I am here to help you redefine your body.

I have been called the All Star Trainer, a Top 10 Trainer, and LA's Best, and I have personally shaped the perfect bodies of Madonna, Demi Moore, Naomi Watts, Sharon Stone, Christy Turlington, and Alicia Silverstone. Now, along with Laurel House, I am going to sculpt your body into its perfect Star Quality shape, too.

Star Quality is a results-driven, celebrity-tested, businesswoman- and stay-at-home-mom-approved fitness and food program that will help you attain long-term goals fast—if you just follow my lead.

I am sure you have heard way too many actresses, models, singers, and celebrity socialites swear, "I don't exercise and I can eat whatever I want and stay skinny." Yeah. And the world is flat. If you want to shape your body to look like a celebrity's, you will have to work out and eat right. Period.

With guidance, fitness and smart eating aren't that hard to do. The hardest part is having motivation and dedication—in other words, not slacking off, and sticking with the program. I will let you in on the secrets that have helped celebs turn their flabby bodies into the fab bodies you see on-screen. Once you get the basics, we will customize your program. It's kind of like a singer who learns the notes or an actress who memorizes her lines, then builds on them, creating her song or her character. I will teach you the fundamentals, then I will show you how to accessorize your fitness regimen with a little glitz and glam. Glitz and glam added to your basic exercise routine will help you create a constantly evolving, personalized, and gym-free fitness program that will tame your body and shape your ideal Star Quality physique.

Combine the exercise with easy recipes that make eating a fat-burning, muscle-building diet effortless, and you have a program that pretty much guarantees success.

Get ready to give this your all. Know that you will sweat buckets (haven't you read in the tabloids how your favorite celebs—at least those who admit to exercising—work out five days a week for up to three hours a day?). You will push yourself further—both mentally and physically—than you ever have, until that nasty fat finally melts away! And like your favorite celebrity, you will have a goal in mind, a goal that motivates you to go a little longer and push a little harder. For an actress, that goal might be looking sexy on the big screen wearing nothing but short shorts and a bikini top. And don't forget the swarm of photographers documenting stars' every move, plastering their fat days and makeupless moments on the covers of the gossip rags. What goal will make you get up and fight that flab?

If you really want this, if you really want to once and for all be in the best shape of your life, do not even attempt to get by with excuses, because the only person you are hurting and lying to is yourself. I know you want it. Come and get it.

Take-It-Outside Philosophy

You know you should strength train to speed up results and boost metabolism, but the sweat-filled weight room at your local gym isn't your favorite place to flex your muscles. You don't have to depend on the gym to get a good strength workout; all you need is the ability to push your own weight. Why do you think push-ups are so hard? Because you are splitting your entire body weight between your hands and toes. Seated dips, squats, wall sits, step-ups—if you want to engage your muscles and exhaust them to the point of soreness in the morning, try my series of exercises!

The Star Quality Program

With this book, I will arm you with the following:

- A twelve-week weight-loss and muscle-toning program backed by testimonials, stories, and tips from real women, including my A-list celebrity clients.
- A fitness and food regimen outlining the basic essential exercise and diet program.
- The glitz and glam to help you personalize your program according to your ultimate body goals. Glitz-and-glam accessories will come in the form of cardio, resistance, and nutrition tips that will change up your regular routine and prevent redundancy-caused ruts, boredom, and dropout.
- A personalized program that addresses different body types, defined by celebrity body types (Madonna-type, Naomi-type, Demi-type), so that you can tailor the workout to your body-molding goals. There is not just one type of celebrity body; there are several, based on the three different body types that every person falls into. Just as there are three basic body types, there is an array of celebrity body–type goals. Some people may want

the athletic body, others prefer the svelte, and still others want the sexy hourglass physique.

- Take-it-outside techniques. No need to buy a gym membership or expensive exercise equipment; I will show you how you can use your environment as your gym.

- Honest information. I have to warn you, I am a straightforward kind of guy, and so is my approach to fitness and food. If you aren't afraid of a direct, efficient, and effective program guaranteed to generate real results, stick with me. This is not going to be an esoteric experience. Working out and getting in your best physical shape is about staying present in your body (though the mind-body connection will be addressed as well).

- Quick tips that will provide you with fresh facts and ideas that you can put to use immediately, including Celeb Secrets, Get Psyched, On-the-Go Exercise, Food Bite, Accidental Exercise, Essential Elements, Food News, and Up the Ante, plus boxed information on how to tweak and expand upon the basic program to attain your ideal celeb body type.

- Sport-specific exercises for athletes. I will show you movements that will help better your game by targeting underused muscles that actually support your favorite fitness activity, from yoga and tennis to skiing and kayaking.

If you are really ready to get in shape for the long term, *Star Quality* presents the program you've been searching for.

1

The Glitz-and-Glam Workout

What is your idea of the perfect body? I doubt it is the shape of a pear, an apple, a ruler, or an hourglass. Come on, is a fruit or an inanimate object really so enviable that obtaining its shape will force your butt out of bed early every morning to work out? Let's get real here. We want to look like celebrities! If you truly want to reshape your physique to star superiority, you have to create a reasonable and attainable goal.

We all have celebrities whom we admire and whose bodies we consider to be perfect. What celeb embodies that perfection to you?

Do you want Madonna's quintessential athletic body? What about Naomi Watts's trim and slim dancer-type body? Or do you aspire to Demi Moore's slender yet voluptuous movie-star body? Those bodies aren't born; they are made. Lucky for you, I have worked with each of those women, and I will reveal their fitness secrets to you.

Before addressing chiseling or slimming, I will pare down exercise to its most basic form. Once the basics are established, we will accessorize your routine with a celebrity favorite—glitz and glam—an extensive selection of five-minute strength-training and fat-burning moves to personalize your program in the ultimate creation of your ideal Star Quality body. Each move targets a specific body part and caters to the specific body type that you were born with. The celebrity body types will serve as examples (in place of the overused and unappealing fruit analogy) to help you focus your attention and achieve your goals. The fact is that just like you, each of your favorite stars was born into a specific shape. Then she took her natural beauty and perfected it with exercise and healthy eating. You can, too.

Honing in, paring down, and focusing is the best way to obtain results fast. I will give you the tools, but I am not going to do all the work.

Putting the "Work" Back in "Workout"

Do you want to know a secret about the business of being a star? Stars are, in part, paid to look good. That's why they pay me to make them look good. How, exactly, do I turn a flabby actress into a leading lady? I make her work—hard!

The average exerciser plateaus after six months because her workout is no longer challenging her body. Muscles learn to expect certain types of repetitive movements if we do them over and over again for months at a time. That's why, within a few months, a really hard routine becomes easy—the muscles are trained. You have taken the "work" out of "workout," allowing the routine to become too easy. That's called cheating . . . cheating yourself.

Adding an extra set of stairs or stepping up your leisurely stride and turning it into a jog or a run is hard—believe me, I hear it all the time. No one wants to do what's hard. No one wants to force herself to do something she isn't good at. Well, guess what? When it's hard, that's when you know it's working—you're working and your muscles are finally being challenged enough to create change.

I am not here to coddle you. I am here to hold up a mirror so that you can really take a good hard look at yourself, at your body, and at what you have let yourself become; then I am going to guide you along a path to change, teaching you the proper, most efficient, and most effective way to work out.

Still with me? Or are you okay maintaining your current body? I know you are ready to change. You wouldn't have picked up this book if you weren't. Follow me and I will show you how. In the next part of this chapter, I'll discuss the three main concepts that you must maintain throughout your training in order to succeed: commitment, consistency, and consciousness.

Commitment

This is a commitment that you are making to yourself. Why is it that when we make a commitment to someone else we stick to it no matter what, but commitments that we make to ourselves we just as soon break? Be honest with yourself about what it's going to take to truly commit to a program that, if you stick with it, will result in serious weight loss, muscle strength, and reshaping of your body.

Is your child your motivation to finally get fit? Or is it a specific goal—like a high school reunion, your first triathlon, or your wedding?

What's it going to take to stick with the commitment to lose that fat? Do you need a partner? Someone who will be waiting for you at the corner at 7 a.m. and will be disappointed if you ditch her because you wanted to snooze through your alarm? If a partner is an essential element, you aren't alone. Why do you think celebrities hire me? Yes, I teach them new techniques and help them focus on the type and amount of cardio and strength training they need to achieve their particular goals. But more than that, they pay me to force them out of bed and onto the pavement. I am there to motivate them through the tough spots and to rouse every last bit of strength until they burn their butts off and are small- and big-screen ready.

Consistency

New behaviors are reinforced and formed into habits through consistency. Keep up with your program. Maintain your routine. Decide on a time of day to exercise that realistically works in your schedule. Then do it. Be consistent.

You won't start shedding that fat and find success if one day you work out for two hours, take the next three days off, then pull yourself back together and power through another excessively long session, followed by a pizza-party celebration and a week off from exercise. You have to maintain consistency, develop a routine, and stick to your program every day.

Consciousness

Are you present? Right now? Or are you just reading along without actually paying attention, kind of like what you do when you are working out? You get on that treadmill, position your magazine on the plastic prop, and dive into the fashion, gossip, and sex tips. You work out for an hour, barely break a sweat, and feel a false sense of triumph. The problem with that too-common scenario is that you paid more attention to the magazine and staring at the sinewy celebrity bodies that fill its pages than you did to your own body. Yes, your legs were moving beneath you, but your mind wasn't in it and, therefore, you weren't working as hard as you could have.

If you are going to commit to an hour of physical activity, take full advantage of that time and work off your weight. Don't waste your time and don't waste mine. I can guarantee that I won't waste yours. Bringing consciousness to your workout means being present and aware of what state your body is currently in and how it feels when you move it and work it. You have to be honest with yourself.

Since I am not there to assess your body's level of strength and endurance, I am depending on you to honestly judge yourself. Show up—mentally and physically—or go home and stay in the shape that you are in.

Fitness Philosophy: Change It Up to Keep It Up

If you want a surefire way to fail a fitness program, do the same workout every single day. If you want to keep up your exercise regimen and get results long term, you've got to change it up. You will experience more change with change.

Physically, changing your daily program keeps your muscles guessing and maximizes your calorie burn. Think about it: walking forward is easy. Moving your legs and arms forward—one foot after the other, swinging your arms in rhythm—has become so easy you could (and some of you do) do it in your sleep. But lifting your legs side to side and pumping your arms up and down forces you to expend more energy, break a sweat, and burn more calories faster.

Mentally, when the movements are constantly changing, you are forced to actually think about what you are doing instead of robotically going through the motions with your mind on something else.

Over fifty glitz-and-glam exercise options will allow you to do a different program every day. By keeping your program varied, you work your entire body while also honing in on problem areas, not to mention the heightened metabolism and heart rate and the maximum calorie burn you'll achieve. So keep going with me!

Define Your Star Quality Body Type

What do you think your celebrity body type is? It might be hard to decipher right now if your body is padded with pudge that hides your sexy shape. But once you cut that fat, your Star Quality body will be revealed! First let's discuss the basics, then we will determine your body type.

Body Basics

There are three basic body types that everyone fits into: ectomorph, endomorph, and mesomorph. Because I find those terms too scientific in tone and, honestly, a bit boring, I am changing them to describe the body types we can actually relate to—those of celebrities. From now on, I will refer to ectomorphs as Naomi-types (as in Naomi Watts), endomorphs as Demi-types (as in Demi Moore), and mesomorphs as Madonna-types (as in Madonna). Let me remind you that these celebs seriously sweat to sculpt their bodies, maximizing their natural potential. You may have excess fat surrounding your Madonna-type figure, but that doesn't mean that you can't slim down, tone up, and develop that type of body that you want.

The Naomi-Type

Naomi-types tend to be thin and linear and often have narrow waists, hips, and shoulders. They easily lose weight but find it difficult to gain muscle and appear toned. Naomi-types are more likely to put on weight in their stomachs and butt while their arms and legs stay slim.

When Naomi Watts and I first started working together, we had two weeks to tone her body to bikini perfection in preparation for a starring role. Naomi appeared to have the ideal body. She was already slim and had a petite, feminine shape. We focused on defining her waist and thighs, refining her rear, and firming her overall physique. Naomi was very much your typical ectomorph—long and lean. We worked less on slimming than on toning and creating feminine curves.

Unlike other body types, Naomi-types don't struggle as much with bulk. They don't need to work as intensely to sculpt their shape. A Naomi-type program is more focused on the basic routine and less dependent on the extra glitz and glam that other body types will need to accessorize with. Excessively long cardio sessions are unnecessary since Naomi-types are already thin. The focus, instead, is on redistributing their body composition, which can actually contribute to weight (not fat) gain because muscle weighs more than fat (muscle also naturally burns more calories than fat).

The Demi-Type

Demi Moore, an hourglass endomorph, is sexy and voluptuous, but she was curvy, and we needed to redistribute some of her weight. Demi knows that part of her job as an actress is to physically fit her film roles. Unlike other actresses who play a specific part when it comes to body type and shape, Demi is known to transform herself, reinventing her body and resculpting her physique on a regular basis. You have seen her body evolve from ripped with muscle for *G.I. Jane* to curvy and cut for *Striptease* and superslim and trim for *Charlie's Angels: Full Throttle*, not to mention perfectly poised and athletic when she posed in the buff on the cover of *Vanity Fair* during the third trimester of her second pregnancy. Postpartum, Demi was dedicated to shedding her baby fat (though there wasn't too much to trim since she stayed active throughout her pregnancy). We wanted to define her waist, and to do that, we decided to accentuate her shoulders, creating a V-shape.

Demi did intense cardio and strength-training sessions on a regular basis. To maintain her interest and avoid making her daily workouts routine to the point of boredom, we explored all the possibilities that her outside environments offered. From snowshoeing during the winter to wading across rivers during the summer, Demi made sure that her workouts were fun. In fact, she often involved her friends, making her workouts group activities that were filled with equal parts sweat and laughter.

The Madonna-Type

Madonna-types have an athletic build. Those with pear-shaped bodies are generally Madonna-types. Madonna-types have broad shoulders and a narrow waist. They gain muscle mass easily and have a fast metabolism, allowing them to lose weight more easily than Demi-types. Madonna-types often have larger lower bodies and smaller upper bodies, with small chests, flat stomachs, and a tendency to gain weight in the hips.

Today, Madonna has a kick-ass body. But that's because she works harder than anyone I have trained at sculpting and maintaining. She is considered a mesomorph, which means she naturally takes on an athletic shape. When Madonna and I started working together, she needed to get in shape for a world tour. Talk about a stressful short-term goal! If you're nervous about impressing a hundred wedding guests or old high school friends, think about what Madonna was going through knowing that millions of fans and critics had microscopes focused on her body and were about to watch her shake her booty on stage—an image that, of course, would be exaggerated on video screens and eternally frozen in photographs.

Madonna maintained a full-throttle intensity day in and day out. She survived grueling workouts that included running for seemingly endless miles (I was running right along with her) up hills—sometimes sidestepping half the way with a jog for recovery, no walking—thirty- to forty-mile bike rides, climbing upwards of thirty flights of stairs. And that was just the cardio. The goal was to increase her oxygen intake so that she could perform more efficiently— singing and dancing with minimal exhaustion and without being out of breath. She did forty-five minutes of strength training with an emphasis on legs. After our workouts, she performed for two hours, four nights a week. She was a world beater!

CELEB SECRETS

Working Out Is Part of the Job

Hollywood casting directors are arguably just as concerned with an actress's body as with her body of work. Why do you think stars have personal training as part of their contracts? Intense daily workouts are as important as acting classes.

What's Your Celebrity Body Type?

What celeb body type are you? Take this quiz to find out! Put a checkmark next to the answers that most accurately describe you.

1. My bone structure is:
   - _____ A. very large
   - __✓__ B. large to medium
   - _____ C. small to frail

2. My body is naturally:
   - __✓__ A. fat
   - _____ B. lean and muscular
   - _____ C. too skinny

3. My body is shaped:
   - _____ A. like a pear—bigger on bottom and lean on top
   - __✓__ B. like an hourglass—balanced on top and bottom
   - _____ C. like a ruler—skinny and straight up and down

4. When I was younger I was:
   - _____ A. overweight
   - __✓__ B. normal
   - _____ C. skinny

5. My activity level is:
   - __✓__ A. nonexistent
   - _____ B. pretty active
   - _____ C. very active, almost antsy

6. My approach to life is:
   - _____ A. relaxed
   - _____ B. dynamic
   - __✓__ C. stressed

7. My metabolism is:
   _√_ A. barely moving
   ____ B. fine, not great
   ____ C. too fast

8. Friends and family who are honest with me tell me:
   ____ A. I should work out and diet
   _√_ B. I look fine and shouldn't change
   ____ C. I am too thin and should gain weight

9. If you encircle your wrist with your other hand's middle finger and thumb, you notice that your:
   ____ A. middle finger and thumb do not touch
   _√_ B. middle finger and thumb barely touch
   ____ C. middle finger and thumb overlap

10. When it comes to weight gain, I:
   ____ A. easily put on weight but have a hard time losing it
   _√_ B. gain and lose weight reasonably easily, but I tend to maintain
   ____ C. have a hard time gaining weight

11. I am hungry:
   _√_ A. almost all the time
   ____ B. only at mealtimes
   ____ C. rarely, not even really at mealtimes

12. I am often described as:
   _√_ A. emotional
   ____ B. physical
   ____ C. intellectual

Now it's time to tally your answers.
For each "A" answer, give yourself 1 point.
For each "B" answer, give yourself 2 points.
For each "C" answer, give yourself 3 points.

Add up all your points and divide the total by 12. Match your score with the body type below.

1 = Demi-type

2 = Madonna-type

3 = Naomi-type

If your total number is a decimal (1.1, 1.9, 2.3, and so on), then you are between two body types (obviously, if you scored 1.8, you are closer to a 2 than a 1) and should focus your workout to your main type, while trying out a few moves for your secondary type, too.

Celebrity-Tested Tips

1. Clearly define your objectives.
   Set up goals based on what you are trying to accomplish. Define why are you starting an exercise program. Redefine your objectives on an ongoing basis.

2. Set up your workout schedule for the week and write it down.
   This is an excellent way to commit to your program and will keep you accountable.

3. Keep workout times consistent.
   This will help establish consistency and long-term success.

4. Make adjustments to your workout based on how you are feeling.
   Some days you will feel good and some days you won't. Always listen to your body.

5. Mix up your workouts.
   This will increase your improvement by challenging your body to adapt to new moves.

6. Follow these tips for proper recovery.
   Consume enough calories to fuel your body. Food is fuel.
   Make sure to get enough sleep.

Keep activity low to moderate outside of your training.

Keep stress levels reduced throughout the day.

7. Exercise with a partner or a friend.

   This will help with consistency and long-term success with the added benefit of motivating each other.

8. Reward yourself.

   When you accomplish a goal or master a new exercise, reward yourself with something special.

9. Listen to music.

   This helps pump you up.

10. Do your personal best on any given day.

    This says it all!

3

What Does Overweight Mean?

So what is cellulite? And how is it different from fat? If you understand the causes, you may be able to change the effects. First let's look at the facts about fat.

Fat

When you eat more calories than you burn, your body stores those excess calories and turns them into fat. We are a nation of overeaters and under-exercisers. It's time to reverse that trend and start to get our bodies back!

How Much Is Too Much Body Fat?

Men generally carry less fat than women because men don't need the extra body fat for childbearing purposes. A healthy man should have less than 18 percent body fat, while women are able to get away with

23 percent or less to be considered healthy (this doesn't mean that women can eat more than men in order to get to that 23 percent; in fact, women tend to gain weight more easily and find losing weight more difficult). According to doc-

Accidental Exercise

Stand Up

Slim people statistically stand for two hours a day, which can burn up to 350 additional calories.

tors, a woman isn't in danger of becoming morbidly obese until she gets up to 40 percent body fat, but she can encounter health problems if she goes over 23 percent.

What Is Body-Fat Percentage?

It is not uncommon for two people who are the same height and weight to have different body-fat percentages. Here's why: the body is made up of fat, tissues, muscle, bone, organs, blood, and lots of water. Your body-fat percentage is your percent of weight from fat. Everything else is called lean body mass. In other words, a 140-pound person with a body-fat percentage of 25 is made up of about 35 pounds of fat and 104 pounds of lean body mass. But another 140-pound person might have only 18 percent fat because she is made up of more muscle than fat. How much body fat compared to lean body mass are you carrying around? Before beginning an exercise and weight-loss program, it is important that you know how much body fat you have.

When losing weight, you want to preserve as much lean body mass as possible. You don't want to get thin while simultaneously getting fat. What I mean is, you don't want to eat such a small amount and not exercise to the point that you get skinny but lose muscle—you'd be a skinny fat person. A skinny fat person may look thin, but maintaining a body like that is very hard to do (not to mention that it is extremely bad for you) because you don't have muscles to burn extra calories during off-exercise hours. Basically, you aren't allowed to eat much of anything in order to stay skinny fat.

What Is the Difference Between Essential Fat and Excess Fat?

You have to carry around some fat on your body in order to function normally. We need fat for insulation, to store energy, to produce and maintain healthy hormone levels, and to cushion our tissues. We naturally store some good fat in the marrow of our bones, and in the tissue of our heart, lungs, liver, spleen, kidneys, intestines, muscles, and central nervous system. We also store some essential fat in the form of deposits (that's what we see as fat on our body). Women store an extra 9 percent body fat for childbearing and hormonal function.

When women don't have enough fat in their essential body-fat stores, they can dip into the childbearing and hormonal stores, which is why a very thin woman might not have a regular period and could temporarily or even permanently risk her ability to conceive. Keep in mind that a healthy portion of a woman's fat is there to support reproduction. Breasts are made up of almost all fat. Women also need fat around their hips. That fat is normal and natural—that is, until you start piling on extra fat on top of that essential fat.

As you age, you might notice that you gain more fat. Your muscles tend to shrink, so that you are naturally burning fewer calories. Hormone levels begin to decrease. This is all natural. What isn't natural is excess fat. Excess fat is the fat that you don't need—the fat that bulges from your belly, thighs, arms, and behind. That is what we are trying to burn off.

How Can I Lose Excess Fat?

The only way to lose excess fat is to burn more energy than you consume (remember that calories convert to energy, which converts to fat if in excess). Your body naturally burns calories throughout the day. Everything you do—from getting out of bed in the morning to cooking dinner, sitting on the couch, even sleeping—burns calories. Women burn between 1,200 and 1,700 calories each day without doing anything. You burn even more calories through exercise.

How Does Exercise Affect Body Fat and Weight?

In addition to burning fat naturally, exercise will increase your muscle mass, which will, in turn, amplify your calorie burn even when you are not exercising. The more exercise you do, the more calories you will burn.

The problem here is that many exercisers feel that since they are working out more, they can eat more to "support" the new fitness program and make sure there are enough calories to be burned. Often they end up eating more calories than they are burning, and they wonder why they aren't losing weight! You really don't need that much more fuel. Eat because you feel hungry, not because you think you should feel hungry.

Why Am I Gaining Weight in My New Exercise Program?

When you first start a workout program, you may actually gain pounds! But don't worry and don't let it discourage you. What is happening is that your muscles are increasing in size and you still have the fat layer over the muscle. Once those new muscles really start pumping and calories start naturally burning away, you will notice that your fat starts to burn off and you will start to look toned and lean.

Why Do We Seem to Gain Weight in the Same Places?

Your body is predisposed to gain fat in certain areas based on your body type and your family's fat history. One common place where women gain fat is in the thighs and hips, while men are more prone to gain weight in their stomach.

Can I Burn Fat from a Specific Spot?

No. But you can tone and tighten specific areas. You might notice that you seem to lose fat in a particular area first—say your face or your arms. When you burn fat, you are burning fat equally from your entire body. It just might be more quickly noticeable in some areas than others.

How Many Calories Do I Need to Burn to Lose One Pound of Fat?

In order to lose one pound of fat, you need to burn approximately 4,000 calories. That's why the concept of losing twenty pounds in one month is nearly impossible. That would equal around 80,000 calories burned. The average woman burns about 700 calories running for one hour. To burn 80,000 calories in one month you would need to run at full speed for 112 hours. That's almost four hours of running each day. You can, on the other hand, lose a lot of water weight in a month. But that is only temporary. Drink a couple cups of water and it will come back. If you want to lose weight long term, you have to burn fat.

Can a Steam Room or a Sauna Help Me Lose Weight?

Technically, yes, you can lose weight in a steam room or a sauna. But you will gain it all back as soon as you rehydrate. Excessive sweating makes you lose water weight, which is very different from fat weight. A similar thing happens when you go on a detox diet that includes diuretics (which force you to lose water weight). You may look leaner for a little while, but it is only temporary. Here's the kicker: when you get out of the steam room and you replace that water loss with a calorie-filled drink, you are actually contributing to weight gain! Believe me, there is no way around it. If you want to lose fat, you have to up your calorie burn through a healthy food and fitness program.

Cellulite

Orange-peel skin. Cottage-cheese thighs. Rippled dimples. Sacks of fat. Over 90 percent of women have cellulite. And contrary to popular belief, this "skin condition" is unbiased, affecting women of all shapes and sizes—skinny, average, and overweight. Believe me, even supermodels and actresses secretly obsess about the cellulite on their thighs, hips, butt, lower belly, arms, and ankles.

If you are unsure as to what cellulite is exactly, let me clarify it for you: fat and cellulite are not one and the same. Cellulite isn't necessarily an abundance of fat. Cellulite is a skin problem that involves fat. Technically, cellulite is free-floating fat cells that have escaped through a weakened layer of connective bands of fibrous muscle tissue made of collagen and elastin that look a little like lace. When the "lace" gets loose, fat is able to seep through, finding its way just below the surface of the skin, where it gets trapped. Once the fat is stuck, it forms the dimples that we call cellulite.

Connective bands weaken because of genetics, age, circulation, and hormones. But hormones are the most common cause of the condition—which is the reason men are rarely affected by it. If you have the hormone levels that cause cellulite to bubble up below the skin, it is likely thanks to genetics. The environment further amplifies the problem in the form of free radical damage caused by too much sun exposure, chemicals in the air, pollution, and other toxins. These toxins need to be filtered out once they seep into your body before they lodge themselves into your tissues and cause or worsen cellulite. And then there's age. Cellulite is superficially a cosmetic problem, but more than that, it is a medical problem that worsens as we get older.

Though cellulite is defined, doctors haven't been able to come up with a surefire cure for it. But you can slow its spread and minimize its appearance by strengthening slackened tissues.

If you are among the 90 percent of women who have cellulite and you want to treat it, you need to heal, strengthen, and hydrate the cells and connective tissues in your body with exercise, diet, and topical products.

- *Exercise.* Regular exercise encourages better circulation throughout the body and in the skin. Spot-specific toning exercises can also strengthen your tissues, helping to firm up the skin and minimize the appearance of cellulite. Losing weight reduces your surface area, making the space that cellulite can encompass much smaller and making its appearance less noticeable.

- *Diet.* Certain foods and supplements can help strengthen connective tissues, repair cell damage, and improve circulation. For example, egg yolk is filled with lecithin, which is said to help move fat. Berries contain antioxidants, amino acids, and anti-inflammatories, which can help regulate cellulite's spread.

- *Hydration.* As we age, our bodies lose some of their ability to properly digest water. Instead of settling into the cells, much of the water we drink either goes right through us or sits in empty spaces between the tissues and cells, causing the appearance of bloating— eyes get puffy and legs and ankles swell. Dehydrated cells struggle to function at their optimal level as they weaken and become deteriorated. When the connective tissue bands lose strength, fat cells (which are attracted to water) more easily slip through and, again, push up against the skin as cellulite. When cells are rehydrated, water shifts back into them, the connective tissue gains some strength, and the freely floating fat cells are less noticeable.

- *Topical solutions.* Several spas swear that for $50 to $5,000 they can make your cellulite disappear. That's because they are using topical treatments, combined with massage and other techniques, to reduce its appearance. Scrubs, wraps, and mud treatments use natural ingredients to help stimulate collagen, encourage circulation, and minimize fluid retention. You can do some of the treatments at home for much less money just by going out and buying the active products. What ingredients help and how?

  - *Caffeine.* Caffeine perks up your mind and body when you drink it. Rub water-soaked grinds on your body and it also gets fluid flowing in your skin, temporarily minimizing cellulite's appearance. You will notice that caffeine is an ingredient in many anticellulite body washes, scrubs, and creams.

- *Seaweed and algae.* The ocean's nutrient-rich ingredients have been used to heal for thousands of years. Seaweed and algae are both filled with minerals can firm and tighten the skin, while slightly plumping the surface area, therefore filling in the pitted spaces along the surface of your skin. This makes cellulite less noticeable.
- *Lecithin and fatty acids.* Lecithin (found in egg yolk) and essential fatty acids (found in flaxseeds, fish, and nut oils) help repair cells and their connective tissues, minimizing fat's ability to squeeze through.
- *Cayenne or chili pepper.* Like caffeine, cayenne and chili pepper help improve circulation, encouraging cell turnover and improving the skin, making it appear smoother and softer.

You can't ignore the fact that your bottom half (and the bottom half of many women—even thin ones) is often heavier than your top half. It seems that the fat cells in your legs and butt are better at hanging on for dear life than those in your arms are. That's because fat cells on your butt and thighs are six times stronger and more resilient, which also makes them harder to get rid of. But it isn't impossible. You just have to fight the good fight and work harder to burn them off.

Cellulite varies in degree. A scale has been created, called the Nurnberger-Muller Scale, to determine how sticky your situation is. Cellulite is most noticeable when you are standing. To figure out how you rate, stand naked in a brightly lit room, face away from a full-length mirror, and look back over your shoulder. Use the following Nurnberger-Muller Scale to figure out just how dimpled your skin has become. The four-stage scale starts at stage 0 (cellulite-free skin) and progresses to stage 3 (severe, painful cellulite).

Stage 0: Cellulite Free

You know you are truly cellulite free if when you stand on your feet or lie on your back you don't see any dimpling, not even when you pinch your skin between two fingers.

Stage 1: Mild Cellulite

If you stand on your feet or lie on your back and there is no visible dimpling, but doing the pinch test causes your skin to ripple, you have mild cellulite.

Stage 2: Moderate Cellulite

If standing reveals cellulite visibly pushing through to your skin, which is only made worse when you pinch your skin between your fingers, but when you lie on your back the rippled dimples seems to go away, you have moderate cellulite.

Stage 3: Severe Cellulite

When standing on your feet and lying on your back naturally expose cellulite, you have severe cellulite. This type of cellulite can actually hurt when touched. Even sitting can be painful as you smash the rogue fat cells against the chair, creating more pressure between your skin and the connective bands that the fat cells escaped from.

If you want a chance at minimizing cellulite's unattractive appearance on your skin, you have to start working out and maintaining a healthier lifestyle right now. Losing weight will pull your skin taut as fat is redistributed and melted away. With less fatty deposits hiding just skin deep, cellulite's appearance will be minimized and you will be free to show off your thighs again.

So let's move!

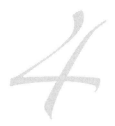

Your Star Quality Fitness Plan

Whether you are a career woman, a stay-at-home mom, or an actress, regardless of your fitness level, you are starting from scratch with this new plan. You are laying a foundation to take your program and your body in a different direction. Within this first month you will be setting realistic short-term and long-term goals for yourself.

Where to begin? Well, you begin where you are right now. Your fitness level is different from my fitness level or your best friend's fitness level. Before you actually start to move your body you need to determine what that level of fitness is. After a series of questions and tests you will know exactly where you stand (that is, if you are honest with yourself—which I require from all of my clients). From that place of awareness and knowledge you will be able to more efficiently and effectively lose fat, gain muscle, and calculate your success.

My system of training allows you to create a comprehensive, constantly evolving program consisting of a basic routine to which cardio and strength training extras are added based on your individual body-type needs. This technique allows you to concentrate on particular muscle groups, reinforcing the movements in order to tone and tighten to your precise specifications.

Once you have your base, you can mix and match, add to your repertoire, and switch focus to another area the next day. This way you can truly sculpt your body like an artist. This method is how personal trainers keep clients interested, motivated, and always seeing change in their bodies. With this book, you have your own personal trainer for a lot less money! What's even better is that no matter where you are—at home, on vacation, even at work—you can get a great workout.

While I show you how to work your body in order to build muscle and burn fat, I will also give you quick tips about what you can do for immediate results. Like this one: cardio has been proven to deflate belly bloat fast. Studies have shown that exercisers who cycle for thirty minutes minimize stomach swelling by 50 percent more than nonexercisers. If that's not a reason to start riding right now, I don't know what is!

During the first two weeks you will be assessing your fitness level. You will need to be aware of how your body is responding to each exercise in order to safely work to your body's potential. That means that you are pushing your body to its limit without crossing over that line to injury. While you don't want to hurt yourself, you don't want to let yourself slack off, either. If after 15 reps you aren't tiring, I will show you how to add extra resistance so that you can effectively work your muscles to momentary fatigue. Doing 100 reps before feeling any fatigue is a waste of your time. If, on the other hand, after 6 reps your muscles are so weakened that they are shaking, I will offer you options to make that exercise easier.

Once you've got the basics down, you will have the freedom to customize your routine to your celebrity body type goal—be it the Demi-type, the Naomi-type, or the Madonna-type.

Assess Your Fitness Level

Part of a trainer's job is to assess where you are physically and emotionally to properly guide you along a personalized path to your perfect body. Because you are there and I am here, I am trusting you to do my job—with my guidance—and assess yourself. If you want to get everything you can out of me and this book, you need to be completely honest with yourself when you do the following tests to figure out your strengths and weakness in everything from what mentally motivates you to what physically challenges you. My point isn't to break you—it is to push you to a point of success.

Let's face it, cheating is only lying to yourself—which isn't going to do me any harm, but it could do some serious damage to you. If you amp up the numbers that reflect your push-up ability or cardiovascular stamina, I will start you at a level that is too difficult for you right now. If the challenge far surpasses your ability, you will either give up because it's too hard or injure yourself because you refuse to give up. Both of these outcomes would be the unfortunate result of a stupid choice. So instead of regretting either scenario, just be honest with yourself and with me and let's get to work at your starting point.

Medical Evaluation

As you would when undertaking any new exercise program, you should consult your doctor before we get started. You might have a condition that could require you to pace yourself, monitor your heart rate, or back off altogether. Being informed is safer than potentially jeopardizing your health by jumping into something and finding out after the fact that you should have taken it easy. An average preworkout checkup is like a basic physical, consisting of an evaluation of your weight, blood pressure, cholesterol, blood sugar, and basic medical and family history. Your doctor will advise you if the Star Quality food and fitness program is right for you.

Fitness Evaluation

Being acutely aware of your physical fitness level—knowing exactly how many reps you can take, how much weight you can hold, how far you can run before your energy wanes—will show me, through you, how much your body can actually endure.

You could very well find that you are stronger than you thought in some areas and weaker in others. And that's normal. You aren't a well-oiled, perfectly balanced machine . . . yet. Being aware of your fitness level will let you know what is too much, too little, and just right.

Work to the level that is enough to strengthen your body without injury. If after a week you feel as if you can push a little harder, as if you are progressing faster than the program I put you on—fantastic! You might have strength that develops and emerges faster than expected.

If, on the other hand, you feel as if you aren't progressing as fast as I am pushing you to advance, slow down. You know your body better than anyone else. Listen to it and you will succeed in this program.

The Fitness Test

This is a standardized self-assessment test used by trainers and doctors around the country to pinpoint a person's level of physical strength. If you are a healthy adult without any physically restrictive disabilities, this test will accurately determine your fitness level. It is not a competition; it is not a race. You are not being judged. Move to your body's ability and record your results.

Arm Strength Test: Push-up

You have probably been doing push-ups in fitness tests since grade school. They are a good judge of arm strength. Women tend to have less arm strength than men. Don't get frustrated. Follow the proper position and do as many push-ups as you can. If you can't do a standard push-up, try the bent-knee push-up. Eventually you should be able to work your way to the standard method.

STANDARD PUSH-UP

Equipment needed   Mat

- Lie on the ground facedown on a mat.
- Place your hands on the ground beside your shoulders with your fingers pointing forward.
- Fold your feet under so that the bottoms of your toes are the only part of your feet on the ground.

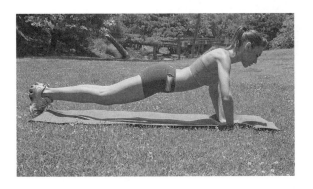

- Inhale, then as you exhale, push your body straight up (do not let your back flex—maintain a straight line along your body) until your elbows are no longer bent, distributing your weight equally between your hands and toes. Do not let your butt sag or poke up.

- Now slowly allow your elbows to bend and with control, lower your body about 6 inches to the point where your forearms and upper arms create a 90-degree angle, and your body is hovering over the ground.
- Repeat.

If you cannot push your body up without arching your back, you should try the bent-knee push-up for now.

BENT-KNEE PUSH-UP

Equipment needed   Mat

- Start on all fours on a mat with your back flat and parallel to the ground, your arms slightly bent to avoid locking your elbows, and your hands placed flat on the ground 2 inches wider than your shoulders and with your fingers pointing forward.
- Your weight should be equally distributed between your hands and knees. Do not let your butt sag or poke up.

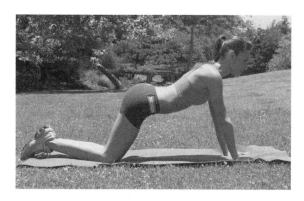

- Slowly allow your elbows to bend and with control, lower your body about 6 inches to the point where your forearms and upper arms create a 90-degree angle, and your body is hovering over the ground.
- Repeat.

How many push-ups were you able to do? Refer to the following chart to assess your results.

NUMBER OF PUSH-UPS							
Age	Excellent	Good	Above Average	Average	Below Average	Poor	Very Poor
17–19	Over 35	27–35	21–27	11–20	6–10	2–5	0–1
20–29	Over 36	30–36	23–29	12–22	7–11	2–6	0–1
30–39	Over 37	30–37	22–30	10–21	5–9	1–4	0
40–49	Over 31	25–31	18–24	8–17	4–7	1–3	0
50–59	Over 25	21–25	15–20	7–14	3–6	1–2	0
60–65	Over 23	19–23	13–18	5–12	2–4	1	0

Abdominal Strength Test: Crunch

Equipment needed   Mat   Masking tape

There are tens, possibly even hundreds, of types of crunches and sit-ups that challenge your abdominals in different ways. To test the core strength of your abdominal muscles, I want you to do just one type, over and over and over until you can't bear to crunch up even once more. Be sure you are in the correct position to avoid injury. Here are the instructions for the crunch I want you to do:

- Lie flat on your back on a mat with your arms at your sides.
- On both sides of your body, stick a strip of tape on both sides of the mat where your fingers end.

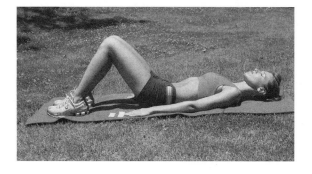

- Place another strip of tape 3 inches past each of the first strips (you will have to sit up slightly to reach this point).
- Now lie flat on your back again.
- Bend your knees and place your feet flat on the ground, allowing your legs to form a 90-degree angle.

- Lay your arms straight along your sides. Do not bend your elbows (be sure that your fingertips touch the first piece of tape).
- Exhale as you use your stomach muscles (not your neck) to curl your chest, shoulders, and head up slightly from the ground in a sit-up motion. Imagine curling your rib cage up toward your pelvis. Your lower back should remain on the ground. This crunch is a very small but effective move.
- Sit up just until your fingertips touch the second pieces of tape.
- Slowly and with control, relax back down to the ground.
- Repeat until you can't do even one more crunch.

How many times were you able to complete the crunch and touch the second pieces of tape? Refer to the chart below to assess your results.

NUMBER OF CRUNCHES				
Age	Excellent	Good	Average	Poor
Under 35	50	40	25	10
36–45	40	25	15	6
Over 45	30	15	10	4

Leg Strength Test: Squat

Equipment needed   Chair

Squats are a typical test of leg strength, particularly quad strength. You are basically doing the same movement that you would do if you were going to sit down in a chair, but without actually sitting, over and over and over again. You have seen this move done by weight lifters who squat with a heavy weighted bar hoisted across their shoulders to intensify the movement. You will squat using the weight of your upper body bearing down on your legs. Here's how to do a proper squat:

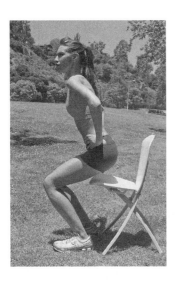

- Find a chair, a couch, or a coffee table that is about knee height.
- Stand with your back to the chair, your feet shoulder-width apart. Do not hold anything in front of you. You will have to use your muscles to balance your body.
- Bend your knees, slightly bend your upper body forward from your waist, stick your butt out, and squat as if you are planning to sit on the seat. *Do not let your butt touch the chair.*
- Once your knees are bent at a 90-degree angle, slowly and with control, stand back up.
- Repeat until you feel the burn in your legs.

How many squats were you able to do? Refer to the chart below to assess your results.

			NUMBER OF SQUATS				
Age	Excellent	Good	Above Average	Average	Below Average	Poor	Very Poor
18–25	Over 43	37–43	33–36	29–32	25–28	18–24	0–18
26–35	Over 39	33–39	29–32	25–28	21–24	13–20	0–20
36–45	Over 33	27–33	23–26	19–22	15–18	7–14	0–7
46–55	Over 27	22–27	18–21	14–17	10–13	5–9	0–5
56–65	Over 24	18–24	13–17	10–12	7–9	3–6	0–3
Over 65	Over 23	17–23	14–16	11–13	5–10	2–4	0–2

Flexibility Test: Seated Forward Bend

Equipment needed   Mat   Yardstick   Masking tape

Some people say that a flexible spine equals a flexible mind. You might say that if you keep your tendons supple, your muscles malleable, and your mind open and active, you will have a long and happy life. Even if you aren't flexible right now, we can work to improve your range of motion and stability. But don't force yourself into a forward bend if your muscles and tendons don't yet have the flexibility to support it. The last thing we want is a tear.

Yes, this is a test. But it is a test to evaluate your flexibility right now. Pushing, pulling, or forcing yourself into positions can result in injury. If you feel any pain at all, stop the exercise immediately. You can come back to this test at a later date once you allow your muscles to recover.

Before you stretch, you must warm up your body for five minutes. Take a walk outside, walk in place, do jumping jacks, swim—do whatever you like. Then let's begin.

- Sit on a mat with your legs straight out in front of you.
- Keep your feet shoulder-width (about 10 inches) apart.
- Place a yardstick between your legs so that one end points toward your crotch area and the other points out beyond your feet.
- The numbers on the yardstick should start small on the end that faces you and get bigger as they move away from you.
- Place your heels on the 15-inch mark.

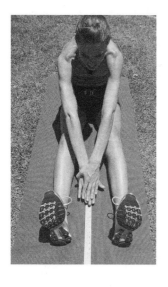

- Tape the yardstick firmly to the mat to hold it in place.
- Stretch your arms out in front of you.
- Place your hands on the ground, one on top of the other. Do not bend your elbows.
- Bend forward at your waist, keeping your back flat.
- Slide your hands along the yardstick as you stretch your torso as far forward as you can. Once you have gone as far as you can, notice the number where the tips of your fingers fall on the yardstick.
- When you think you have reached your limit, take a deep breath and see if your exhale allows you to push just a little bit farther.
- Make a note of that number.

- Repeat this exercise 3 times. You should be able to extend out slightly farther each time.

How far were you able to stretch? Refer to the chart below to assess your results.

EXTENSION IN SEATED FORWARD BENDS, IN INCHES				
Age	Excellent	Good	Average	Poor
20–29	Over 22	16–21	13–15	0–12
30–39	Over 21	15–20	12–14	0–11
40–49	Over 20	14–19	11–13	0–10
50–59	Over 19	13–18	10–12	0–9
Over 60	Over 18	12–17	9–11	0–8

Cardiovascular Endurance Test: Step-Up

Equipment needed   Step, stair, or stool
Heart rate monitor

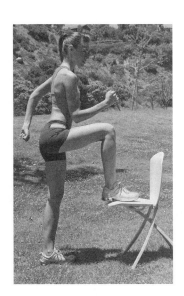

There are several ways to test your cardiovascular endurance—in other words, your heart strength when it is elevated for an extended period of time. Running is one way to push your heart rate. But I like step-ups because you stay in one basic spot, yet you get great results. To do this step-up test you will need a step, a stair, or a very sturdy stool that can support your weight and won't move forward. Your step should not be more than one foot off the ground. Let's start stepping!

- Raise one foot onto the step, then raise your second foot to meet the first. Immediately place your first foot back on the ground, followed by your second foot so that both feet are again on the ground.

- Continue stepping up and down at a steady pace without taking breaks on the step or on the ground.
- Repeat for 3 minutes.
- Immediately after you are finished, check your pulse for one minute. Refer to the chart below to assess your results.

			PULSE RATE				
Age	Excellent	Good	Above Average	Average	Below Average	Poor	Very Poor
18–25	Under 85	85–98	99–108	109–117	118–126	127–140	Over 128
26–35	Under 88	88–89	100–111	112–119	120–126	127–138	Over 138
36–45	Under 90	90–102	103–110	111–118	119–128	129–140	Over 140
46–55	Under 94	94–104	105–115	116–120	121–129	127–135	Over 135
56–65	Under 95	95–104	105-112	113–118	119–128	129–139	Over 139
Over 65	Under 90	90–102	103–115	116–122	123–128	129–134	Over 134

Diet Evaluation

A well-crafted fitness routine is a huge part of a successful weight-loss or weight-management plan. But it's not the entire equation. You have to be aware of your diet. When I say "diet," I don't mean restricting calories for a certain period of time and then going back to your old food ways. I mean making eating well a habit that helps support your fitness. Eating nutritionally balanced meals gives you energy and strength. It can help your body build muscle. It can even stimulate your metabolism. Both building muscle and stimulating your metabolism help you to burn more calories. Eating well can also improve your mood and amp up your immune system.

Long-term nutritional deficiencies can result in serious health problems. Beyond simple weight gain, you are putting yourself at risk for developing cardiovascular disease, diabetes, even cancer. A healthy diet and fitness regimen can greatly reduce your risk of dying young.

To eat well you have to watch portion size, eat frequently (five small meals a day is best to maintain energy and concentration levels) and make good food choices, being aware of vitamins and minerals as well as the balance of proteins and healthy carbs. I will teach you how to maintain a healthy diet that will fuel your fitness program and keep you healthier longer.

To get you started thinking about how nutritionally balanced your diet is, answer the following questions:

Do you watch portion sizes?

Do you drink at least eight glasses of water daily?

Do you check food labels on processed foods?

Do you prepare meals at home with your health in mind?

Do you know how to make healthy substitutions?

Do you focus on eating high-fiber, high-protein, low-fat meals?

Do you eat several servings of fresh fruits and vegetables daily?

Do you keep your intake of sugar to a minimum?

Do you select lower fat, high-quality meats and proteins?

If you didn't answer yes to the majority of questions, you need to rethink your food choices, focusing on being healthy and eating a balanced diet. Yes, it will take some thought and planning. You might have to go out and buy a few items that you have never eaten before. But if you want real results, committing to changing your eating habits will make a huge impact. I know how hard it can be to alter your routine, to give up patterns and preferences that you have had for years, maybe even decades. But believe me when I tell you that you will be happy you did. So you might not be able to eat fast food every night anymore. But isn't waking up filled with energy, breezing past 3 p.m. without feeling like you need to take a nap, and adding five years to your life worth giving up that extra candy bar?

Even if you answered no to just a couple of questions, you have something to work on. Small changes can radically benefit your life in both the short and long term.

Mental Fitness: Test Your Level of Stress

You might be physically fit, but are you mentally fit? In order to successfully change your habits and maintain a healthy lifestyle, you have to be ready for mental challenges as well as physical challenges. Your mind powers your body. When you don't want to stick to your eating and exercise plan because it hurts/because you are tired/because you have hit a plateau/because you really want that piece of cake, your mind will have to keep your body going in a healthy direction.

Mental health and physical health have a lot to do with each other. You have to be mentally fit to force your body to work out when it doesn't feel like it. You have to be physically fit to have a clean mind. Studies show that exercise is one of the most efficient ways to reduce stress. When you come home from a brutal day at work, you might want to eat a big comforting meal accompanied by a hearty glass of wine. If instead you find enough motivation to lace up your running shoes and channel that frustration into a good hard run, or even just a quick sprint at the end of a walk, you will forget why you were so stressed in the first place. Your stress will be replaced with pride for having completed your workout and burned calories. Exercise makes you both physically and emotionally lighter.

> **Accidental Exercise**
>
> ## Just Think!
>
> Don't dismiss the calorie-burning exercise associated with mental function. Thinking can be a calorie-burning workout! Studies show that as much as 20 percent of the energy that your body makes (remember that calorie expenditure equals energy) is consumed by your brain. Not only are mental and physical activities connected, but the food you eat is directly related to your brain—yet another reason to eat a nutritionally balanced diet. Withholding essential nutrients from your diet can affect your brainpower, reducing memory retention and learning ability, trying your patience, and making you more susceptible and reactive to stress.

Understanding Stress

Before I give you your mental stress test, I want you to understand just how serious stress can be. Let me show you the facts:

- According to the Centers for Disease Control, 90 percent of doctor visits each year are to address stress-related health concerns.

- Stress depresses the immune system and can reduce the body's ability to fight free radicals, which can increase your risk of cancer, make you more prone to colds, and increase signs of premature aging.

The severity of stress has in many ways been dismissed in our society. We throw around the phrase "I'm so stressed" like we do "I'm on a diet." To be stressed is almost trendy—as though being stressed makes others perceive us as more successful because we are so overwhelmingly busy with very important things. The problem is that when you say you're stressed enough times, even if you have little to be stressed about, you start to feel the symptoms of stress.

Look, stress isn't a status symbol. The only thing that being in a constant state of stress will do is wear you out, tear your body down, and leave you feeling unnecessarily frenzied.

Let's look at it realistically: what are you really so stressed about? Are you in a desperate race to save the world or save a life? No, you are "so stressed out" because you are ten minutes late to an appointment, you have to finish a project and file a monthly financial report by the end of the week, or you overbooked your business and social lives and have no time for yourself.

As bad as stress may be on our bodies, it actually does serve a very important role—it triggers the fight-or-flight response. Stress is the fuel we know as adrenaline. It is what we called upon during caveman times to help us run from a bear or climb a tree when being chased by an elephant. Stress allows us to tap into our internal energy reserves for short periods of time. The problem with living in an unceasingly stressful society is that our bodies are always required to pull from our reserve energy, demanding that it come to our aid on a regular basis.

Of course, there are those people who say they "thrive on stress." Those people may do better under pressure because they are working with amped-up resources. But when you're not in one of those make-or-break situations, it is essential to let your body rest, restore its reserves, and get ready for the next time you have to defend your territory or run like hell to protect yourself.

One of the many problems with stress is that its symptoms can be hard to nail down. We experience stress in different ways, many of which resemble other ailments like colds, flu, and other viruses. Or we may feel just plain lazy. The reason is that stress lowers the immune response, which therefore makes us more prone to sickness—everything from colds to cancers. Cancer may not be caused solely by stress, but stress can increase your chances of getting cancer. One person might experience stress as a headache (which makes sense considering that when we are stressed we might tense our jaw or shoulders) or a stomachache. Another person might feel anxious and have difficulty sleeping, while someone else might be constantly lethargic and exhausted. Be aware of your body's stress signs and learn to manage them. Exercise is a great option to keep your level of stress in check.

Signs that you are in an unhealthy state of stress can show up physically, mentally, and behaviorally.

Physical signs. Difficulty sleeping, headache, stomachache, muscle spasms (particularly over the eye), exhaustion, rashes, acne breakouts, muscle pain, constant colds or flu, unusual weight gain or loss.

Mental signs. Forgetfulness, apathy, lack of motivation to do anything, depression, anxiety, difficulty focusing, low self-esteem.

Behavioral signs. Moodiness, raging temper, low sex drive, lack of interest in being social, obsessive-compulsive behaviors, alcohol/food/drug addictions, violent behavior.

Your lifestyle, personality, and social tendencies may increase your chances of suffering from unhealthy levels of stress.

Lifestyle. "Hard living"—such as alcohol or drug abuse, an irregular sleep schedule, bad food choices, or inactivity.

Personality. Low self-esteem, being a control freak, perfectionism, obsessive-compulsive disorder, workaholism.

Social tendencies. Lack of friends, lack of support group to vent, difficulty managing conflict.

Don't go around stressing about your need to completely remove stress from your life. Remember, stress helps you to respond quickly in emergency situations (like jumping out of the way of a car), and it also helps you complete and turn in projects with a day's notice. As the endocrinologist Hans Selye once said, "Without stress there would be no life."

The Stress Test

Answer yes or no to the following questions.

- Is your way always the "right" way? NO
- If you want something done, do you have to do it yourself in order for it to be done right?
- Are you constantly giving to others—employer, spouse, children, friends—leaving no time for yourself? Yes
- Do others criticize you by saying that you always have to make a "big deal" out of everything? NO
- Is your physical environment cluttered? NO
- Is your life cluttered? NO
- Do you keep your emotions inside? NO
- Do you put off your fitness routine on a regular basis? Yes
- Do you have an unhealthy diet? Yes
- Do you have unrealistic expectations of people and life? NO
- Do you take everything too seriously? NO
- Do you have a hard time sitting still and relaxing? NO
- Do you depend on sleeping pills or alcohol to fall asleep at night? NO
- Do you have a short temper? NO
- Do you feel as if you never have enough time to get everything done? Yes
- Are you constantly surrounded by loud noise? NO
- Do you frequently experience a racing heartbeat when not exercising?

- Do you have a hard time taking a deep breath?
- Do you feel restless when you try to sit still?
- Do you sweat when other people are cold?
- Do you fixate on small problems that may be insignificant to others?
- Do you have a dry mouth even after drinking water?
- Do you wake up in the middle of the night and can't fall back to sleep because your mind is racing with to-do lists?
- Do you have diarrhea or constipation on a regular basis?
- Are you often nauseated for no reason?
- Do you feel constantly on the verge of crying?
- Do you have a hard time concentrating?
- Have you lost interest in sex?
- Do you feel lonely?
- Are you angry for no reason?

Of these thirty questions, how many did you answer yes to? If you answered yes to half or more, you are experiencing an unhealthy state of stress and you need to focus on doing something to diffuse your stress every day.

If you answered yes to twenty-five or more of these questions, your stress level is a serious concern and you need to talk to a doctor about how you can manage stress.

Ways to Relieve Stress

These are just some of the many things you can do to combat stress.

- Exercise for at least twenty minutes, six days a week.
- Eat healthy, nutrient-rich meals.
- Get on a regular sleep schedule and sleep for enough hours that you wake up energized. (Conventional wisdom says you have to get eight hours of sleep, but everyone is different. If your body functions optimally after six, fine. Listen to your body.)

Runner's High

Exercise has been proven to help minimize stress. More than providing that euphoric feeling from knowing you are working to better yourself, increasing your self-esteem, and achieving mini-goals with every completed session, working out chemically calms you. When you exercise, your blood starts pumping faster through your veins; you take deeper, more cleansing, and detoxifying breaths; and your brain releases endorphins—your body's natural "feel-good" chemicals which some people refer to as "runner's high." In fact, runner's high can last much longer than your actual exercise routine. Some exercisers experience a lightened mood for up to forty-eight hours after the workout session ends.

CELEB SECRETS

Madonna's Tour Schedule

When Madonna was on tour, we trained for two to three hours a day, six days a week! We'd run for an hour to seventy-five minutes or go for a thirty-mile bike ride (yes, I said thirty miles!). This is one woman who is seriously dedicated to both her body and her body of work.

- Create a support group of friends you can confide in.
- Minimize your alcohol intake.
- Stop doing recreational drugs.
- Find ways to release stress—try baths, massage, acupuncture, or meditation.
- Don't overcommit yourself. You don't need to say yes to everyone.
- Alter your mind-set and force yourself to think positively.
- If you don't feel you can manage your stress on your own, ask your doctor for help.

Fitness Philosophy— Take It Outside

Do you have a gym membership? Do you ever use it? How much money have you wasted on unused memberships over the years? If you belong to a gym that you actually go to on a regular basis, how much of your gym time do you spend socializing and slacking off? How about that treadmill that doubles as a clothing hanger in the corner of your room? The best gym doesn't cost a dime; it's in your own backyard—the streets, mountains, beaches, and fields that surround your home.

Another reason to take it outside? Fresh air. I mean really, do you want to suck up sweat-saturated air at the gym? When you take those big inhales, suck up the natural energy of the outdoors. That fresh air and warm sun naturally encourage a kick-butt workout—a much better option than

Get off the Treadmill and Burn More Calories Outside

If you like the treadmill, try pounding the pavement for a change. Running outdoors has been proven to burn more calories and more efficiently tone muscles than doing the same run on a treadmill. Why? The motorized treadmill propels itself, and you, forward, giving you an extra boost. Running outdoors forces you to push yourself forward without the motorized assistance, plus it naturally has a constantly changing incline and decline. Unless you are regularly adjusting the incline on your treadmill, you are not challenging your muscles as you would if you were outside.

the energy-sapping, emotionally depressing artificial lighting in a gym.

Bad weather? Bad excuse to opt out of your outdoor workout (unless, of course, it is a torrential rainstorm or a serious heat wave). Even if it's raining, get outside and run! You aren't going to melt. If Demi and Madonna can run in snow, a little rain won't hurt you; in fact, it can be energizing. You might even run longer since you won't notice how much you are sweating.

Fitness Lifestyle

Like brushing your teeth, taking a shower, even breathing, exercising should be a no-brainer. It isn't just about short-term goals, like fitting into your wedding dress or downsizing for summer; fitness is a lifestyle. Of course, the short-term goals may motivate you to get fit now, but once you attain your target fitness level, you have to maintain, or you will slip back to the beginning and have to start all over again—not fun after all that hard work.

I know, "fitness lifestyle" is a term that is often thrown around. Let me explain. Even the most resistant clients who are night owls, barflies, and party hoppers eventually commit to a fitness lifestyle. Why? Because it feels good to be healthy.

Creating your own fitness lifestyle workout schedule is easy. This is how it works.

- Decide that it is finally time to get your act together and work your butt off (literally).
- Set a goal.

Demi Moore Keeps It Interesting

Demi looked to me to work fitness into her life and keep it from becoming routine. To keep her interested, I kept it interesting. An average summertime week with Demi at her Idaho ranch was as follows:

Monday: hiking

Tuesday: street biking

Wednesday: running

Thursday: kayaking

Friday: mountain biking

In the winter we would take advantage of the snow. One day we might spend an hour and a half snowshoeing, pulling ourselves up a sheer three-hundred-foot incline with a rope, climbing over logs and big rocks, and leaping over rivers. Then we would do resistance work for twenty to forty-five minutes.

- Set your alarm and force yourself out of bed after boozing, bingeing, or simply staying up killing time too late the night before.

- When that alarm goes off, *no snoozing!*

- Get up, put on your running shoes, and hit the pavement (even if it seems painful).

For the first five minutes your eyes will still be struggling to see what's in front of you. Your head may still be foggy. Your body may beg you to turn around and get back in bed. Push yourself to continue—you made it this far, so you may as well keep going. Ten minutes into it, pick up the pace, elevate your heart rate, move blood into your muscles, and begin to break a sweat (let me warn you that if a heavy dose of booze is in your body from the night before, the stench will emanate from your pores—you are detoxing that gunk out . . . it's a good thing). After half an hour your body will be pumped. You will feel more alive than you have felt in a long time. Your brain will buzz and your creative juices will flow. For the rest of the day, even if you are slightly tired, you will be more productive than you have been in months. At night, when it's finally time to go to sleep, you will drift off without the tossing and turning that usually tortures you.

Do this every day, and after a week or so you will begin to feel and see a real difference, not only in your mind and in your life, but in your body. Your skin will seem to be more taut and toned as your muscles tighten and cling to your bones instead of flabbing along with the fat that sits below the surface. You won't want to stay out as late because you know that you will then be tired and less efficient in the morning. You won't want to drink too much or smoke too heavily because you know that it will affect your workout. You won't want to eat that third slice of pizza because you know it will negate the calories burned that morning. You will find friends who want to work out with you and you'll form a buddy system, waking one another up in the morning like personal trainers. They will cheer you on, pump you up, encourage your success, understand your pitfalls, and, of course, keep you company—fitness can be a social event, you know, and a good way to catch up with friends. A few weeks later you will begin to surround yourself with healthier people. The same clothes that used to cling to your skin will soon be hanging from your limbs. You will get more work done faster and live life to a fuller extent. You will experience a renewed enthusiasm for all that you do. I am telling you, this is true. I'm not just blowing smoke. Suddenly you will realize that, yes, you live a fitness lifestyle. Then it's time to get specific.

Target Toning

There is a difference between spot reducing and target toning. You can't spot reduce (shed fat in a particular area), but you can target tone (tighten the muscle in a particular area). Target toning involves bringing awareness to a specific area in order to engage the supporting muscles. Target zones tend to be more difficult to work. Why? Because those areas are weaker and we don't like to work on them since it is hard and painful. We have been trained to place our focus on our strengths. Guess what, ladies—if you want to perfect your body, you have to focus on your weaknesses.

All women (celebrities included) have very specific areas of concern that you can, and we will, target. Let's break them down.

- *Stiletto calves.* Wearing stilettos can put stress on your shins, calves, and ankles. Create a strong and sexy curve along your calf line by doing calf raises.
- *Chest/armpit pudge.* Tube tops that press into your chest can cause the fat that resides beside your armpit and just above your chest to bubble up into a flabby bulge. Even tank tops can accentuate those fatty sacks. Pressing motions, like bench presses and push-ups, can tone and tighten that target zone.
- *"Bat wings"/underarm flap.* Stop saggy arm jiggle by toning up with tricep work.
- *Bra-strap fat.* You know that pudge that protrudes along the top of your bra strap across your back, causing unsightly bulges and wrinkles in tight shirts? You can shed bra strap fat by strengthening your lats.
- *Big butts/flat butts.* Women with big butts will focus on toning and lifting. Those with flat butts will focus on accentuating. In order to attain your goal, you need to exercise in a specific way, essentially doing the same movements, but with different intensity. To downsize your behind, you will want to do my five-minute glute workout with high reps and low resistance. The exercises incorporate aerobic conditioning that focuses on posterior movements to reshape and tone the glutes, hamstrings, and quads in order to lift and lean. To accentuate your assets, you'll want to place more resistance on them. Squats and lunges coupled with specific glute exercises will help to amplify the definition.

Sometimes target toning can be amplified by behavior modification. Standing up straight when you walk will make you appear taller, leaner, and more confident. Sitting up instead of hunching over at your desk will help keep your shoulders back, strengthening your chest and back and even toning your stomach muscles.

Star Quality Body Breakdown

To focus on specific problem areas, you need to know how your body parts break down. I can't just tell you to work your back, because there are a lot of different muscles in your back, and pages of exercises geared to address each area. A spare tire around your waist that spills into your lower back is very different from the roll below your bra strap, which has nothing to do with that extra pocket of pudge at the base of your neck. Familiarizing yourself with a few of the essential muscles throughout your body will make it easier to hone in and tone up!

Let's start at the top and work our way down.

Shoulders

Shoulders work in conjunction with your arms, back, and chest to push, pull, and lift heavy weight. Strong shoulders can completely change your physique. They can make your hips appear slimmer, your waist appear trimmer, and your entire core more balanced and symmetrical. The goal is to make your shoulders as wide as your hips. With broad shoulders, you can have a more statuesque presence. But shoulders that fold forward to meet pudgy arms might not be the eye-catchers you want them to be. If you have narrow shoulders, you can easily add lean muscle mass. If your shoulders lack definition, you can tone and trim them.

Your shoulders are more than the widest part of your upper body; they wrap around to your back into the shoulder blades. The shoulder blades are separated by your spine, which runs down your entire back. Pulling your shoulders back for correct posture requires you to simultaneously focus on pulling your shoulder blades together toward your spine, closing the space between them. The bra-strap fat that puffs out just below your armpit actually sits next to the outside of your shoulder blade. Keeping your shoulder blades close together can help cut that back fat.

Deltoids

The deltoid muscles, also known as the delts, cap the shoulder. They consist of three sections: the anterior, lateral, and posterior delts. The anterior delt and lateral delt muscles begin at the collar bone, just below your neck. The anterior delts assist in any muscle movement of the pecs (the chest), while the lateral delt muscles help maintain sideways movement of the shoulders. The posterior delts originate at the base of the shoulder blades and help coordinate back movements. Work your delts and you will soon be able to proudly display toned shoulders.

Rotator Cuff

The rotator cuff is a group of four muscles that fall along both your back and chest to protect the shoulder joint. A strong rotator cuff is essential for stability. If you have a shoulder injury, the rotator cuff may get the brunt of it. Its susceptibility to various stressors is often due to overuse in incorrect positions. Properly strengthening the muscles of the rotator cuff can help maintain your shoulder's integrity and minimize tension and trauma.

Back

When you get dressed, do you turn around to see what everyone behind you gets to stare at and critique? I have news for you—you should. If you have back fat, as way too many women do, you would be surprised by how bad some tight shirts and tank tops look on you. Fat ripples above, below, and underneath the bra strap, running across your back, forcing the rolls up closer to your armpits or down toward your waist. Believe me, it's not a good look. The average woman spends too much time perfecting mirror muscles—the muscles you see when you are looking at yourself in the mirror—and not nearly enough (if any) on the muscles others see from behind. So either wear a bra that's too big for you and doesn't squeeze your back at all, or do the smarter thing and focus on back exercises. When it comes to target toning, the back is one of the most neglected spots on the body. Following are some of the most important and underworked back muscles.

Trapezius

The trapezius muscles, also known as the traps, are located at the center top of your back on either side of your spine. They travel from mid–shoulder blade level all the way up your neck. Carrying heavy purses or backpacks creates tension on the traps, which can lead to neck tightness, too. In fact, knots in the shoulders are often caused by tight traps. Strengthening those muscles will make lugging around suitcase-size purses less strenuous. Toned traps also help accentuate your shoulders' shape.

While working out your traps, it is important to be aware of how often you call on them to help hoist heavy weight—not a good thing.

The tendency is to displace heavy arm weight by moving some of the tension to your shoulders and using the strength of your traps to power the movement. To avoid a thick weight lifter's neck, keep your shoulders down when working out. Excessively muscular traps can make the neck wide, but perfectly toned traps make the neck appear slim and trim. Having trouble keeping the weight out of the traps? If you feel your neck engage when it shouldn't, slowly turn it right and left. The gentle rotation brings an awareness to the muscles, reminding them to relax.

Rhomboids

The rhomboids are the soft tissues situated between the shoulder blades that tighten up the midback and minimize the appearance of midback bra fat. Rhomboids also help perfect your posture by pulling your shoulder blades together, which assists in standing up straight and tall.

Latissimus Dorsi

The latissimus dorsi muscles, also known as the lats, are the biggest muscles on the back. The lats begin at the side of your waist, then fan up and expand out across your back just below the shoulder blades. Strong lats contribute to a slim waist and assist in just about every torso movement. They help you stabilize your core and maintain control when leaning back or twisting around.

Erector Spinae

The muscles that run along your spine from your tailbone to your skull are called the erector spinae. Strong erector spinae help minimize injury and alleviate lower back pain, from which one-third of Americans suffer. These muscles also contribute to the alignment of your spine and help you maintain your posture.

Chest

So many women wouldn't need to get their breasts lifted if they worked the muscles that support them. Our society has been conditioned to be too blasé about plastic surgery. Ladies, surgery is serious. You pay a bundle of bucks to be put out (which is risky in itself), opened up, and surgically enhanced. My belief is that if you can do it yourself, without the assistance of a surgeon, then get off your butt and do it! Every body part is supported by muscles that can be exercised, strengthened, toned, and therefore lifted. Your breasts are the perfect example. Just as you might exercise your arm muscles, you need to work the muscles below your breasts in order to keep them tight and lifted (which might even make them look bigger).

The pectoral muscles, also called the pecs, consist of the pectoralis major and pectoralis minor muscles that run along the upper half of your rib cage (your breastbone), wrap around your upper side below your armpit, and continue up the front of your shoulder. Because the muscles run across your chest in a fanlike form, they control a full range of multiplanar movement. Strengthening your pecs will help increase your ability to do anything from simply shrugging your shoulders to pushing something heavy away from you. When toned and tightened, the pecs also accentuate the appearance of your breasts, helping to lift them and therefore make them appear firm and full.

Arms

One of the first areas that clients ask me to tone and trim are their arms—especially during tank top and swimsuit season. You want your arms to appear shapely, not stumpy; muscular but not Popeye big. To get Star Quality arms, be sure to focus on all areas of your arms, not just your mirror muscles.

Triceps

The triceps begin just below the back of your shoulders, continue down the back of your arms, and end at your elbows. I wouldn't be exaggerating if I said that every woman I know is, or has been, concerned with their "bat wings"—the flap of skin, fat, and loose muscle that hangs from the back of your arms and shivers when you shake. You might think that flap is pure fat, but it's not. If you stop using the tricep muscles, in time the fibers actually loosen and detach from the bone, causing them to just lie there. Thankfully, you can tighten them back up and have strong triceps with just a little work.

Biceps

The biceps are located in the front of the arm, extending from below the shoulders to the bend at the elbows. They are one of the most recognized and referred to muscles. Think about it. When someone says, "Flex your muscle," what are they asking you to do? Flex your bicep muscle. The most common function of the biceps is to bring your forearm to your shoulder. The second motion that most engages the biceps is turning your hand from facing down to facing up. Biceps are also used to push and pull, carry and pick up. Men tend to have more developed biceps than women. But that doesn't mean they always have to do the heavy lifting. Flex your muscles and carry your own weight!

Abdominals

Having ripples of muscle along the stomach (the "six-pack") is a display of strength and, often, sex appeal. Men tend to achieve this musculature more than women, but you can still shape your abs to be visibly strong and toned. You can trim the tire roll around the stomach and tone your abs to perfection by working out your surface, deep, and side abs.

Rectus Abdominus

Your rectus abdominus is the long sheet of abdominal muscles that starts right below your chest and ends just above your pubic bone. It consists of what many people wrongfully call the "upper" and "lower" abs. Let me make one thing clear here: there is no such thing as upper and lower abs. The abs are the abs. You can target a specific spot of the abs when working the muscle, but you can't isolate the upper from the lower; it is one continuous muscle.

The rectus abdominus is what forms the six-pack abs. It expands when you inhale and contracts when you exhale. Your rectus abdominus helps support your back, taking the brunt of bending, standing, and twisting movements in order to give your back a break. These muscles also contribute to perfect posture.

You may want a flat stomach and you very well will get it. But the reality is that no matter how strong your abs are, in order to have a pouchless stomach you have to lose the fat that sits on top of it. You can do this only by eating healthfully and doing cardio. Once the fat falls away, your cut abs waiting below it will appear.

Internal and External Obliques

Your internal and external obliques are diagonal muscles that wrap around your sides and end at your rectus abdominus. They help you twist your body, stabilizing you so you maintain control. They also help support your back muscles. While your rectus abdominus is in charge of the belly pouch, it is the responsibility of your internal and external obliques to keep your sides from flapping over your jeans.

Transverse Abdominus

Your transverse abdominus is a muscle deep within your abdominal region that acts as a stability belt, cinching your stomach and keeping your insides from falling out. It works to maintain stability and keeps you standing straight and tall.

Butt and Hips

"Butt," "derriere," "ass," "rear," "rump"—there are lots of words to refer to the behind. Now it's time to focus some fitness attention on getting it trim, round, tucked, toned, and slim.

Glutei Maximi

The glutei maximi, also known as the glutes, are some of the largest and strongest muscles in the body; but that doesn't mean they have to be the fattest! Your glutes help you power up stairs, run long distances, jump, and stand. They also serve as a cushion (some bigger than others) for long periods of sitting. If your glutes are weak, you may transfer the work to your lower back and hamstrings. The problem is that if you don't target your glutes during your exercise routine, your butt will begin to sag, get flabby, and lose the sex appeal that it was intended to have. Don't depend on the new "butt bra" jeans that temporarily lift and tighten your behind. If you tone it naturally—with exercise—it will look good when you get out of the shower, too. Work out your glutes and you will also eliminate panty-line bulge (the lines that make it look as if you have four butt

---

CELEB SECRETS

Naomi Watts Toned Up Her "Problem Zones"—Her Abs and Butt

When Naomi and I first started working together, she had concerns about her abs. To up the intensity of her ab workout I always added abs exercises in between sets of other exercises. These extra ab sets served several purposes: they kept her heart rate up, maintained a training pace that maximized caloric expenditure, and further strengthened her abs.

Her other area of concern was her butt. When I first spoke to Naomi, she told me she had to be in a bikini within five days. The short time was a major concern. Thankfully the production crew pushed the bikini scene back two weeks! To firm her glutes, we ran stairs during our cardio work and continued with compound exercises for her lower body. It paid off! Several weeks after filming her bikini scenes she received the trailer for the movie, which featured her in the bikini. We watched the trailer together and she couldn't believe how great her butt looked!

cheeks instead of two), minimize the appearance of cellulite, and burn off your saddlebags. Soon, your ideal Star Quality tush will be revealed!

Hip Flexors

The hip flexor muscles, also known as the iliopsoas, consist of two muscles—the iliacus and the psoas major. The iliacus extends from the pelvic crest to the femur. The longer psoas major is attached on the lumbar vertebrae and ends at the femur. Together they control the movement of the thigh flexing up to the abs and the abs moving down to the thigh (as would happen if you raise your leg or do a sit-up). Overdeveloped hip flexors become tight and can create tension in the lower back, causing your pelvis to tilt. You have to stretch your hip flexors if you want to keep your back and pelvis in balance. You can also counteract the strength by working on the opposing muscles—your abs.

Legs

Show off your shapely gams by toning them up and trimming them down.

Quadriceps

The quadriceps, also known as the quads, are a group of four muscles in the front of each thigh extending from just below the pelvic bone to just above the knee. Their primary responsibility is extending your knees to the straight position; they are also used to climb, run, walk, hop, skate, and ski (notice the size of the quads on pro speed skaters or skiers). Maintaining strong quads will help prevent knee problems. Quads can be very strong and developed since they are used all day to carry you around. For this reason it can also be a challenge to truly feel them burn when working out. It takes a lot of cardio and resistance reps to really activate them and create change.

The vastus medialis is one particular quad muscle that deserves extra attention. This muscle is tear-shaped and it drops down beside the knee. Its function is to support the knee and protect it from injury.

Hamstrings

The hamstrings, also known as the hams, are made up of three muscles that extend from the back of your thighs to the bottom of your glutes. The hams are fast-twitch muscles, which means that they respond best to low reps of heavy weight or powerful movement. The primary focus of the hams is to flex the knees, allowing you to fold your heels to your glutes and push your straight legs back behind you. Hams tend to be vulnerable to pulls and tears because they are usually less developed than their opposing force, the quads. Minimize your chances of injury by warming up your hams before working them and gently stretching them after your workouts. Even casual movements like bending down to pick up something or suddenly running to chase the dog can result in a tear if you have tight hams. You know your hams are tight if you bend forward with straight legs to touch your toes and you feel pain in the back of your thighs—those are your hamstrings.

Calves and Ankles

Having slender, shapely calves that taper into thin ankles (as opposed to tree stumps shooting straight down from your calf muscles into your feet) is important if you want to look good in dresses and shorts. There are several muscles you need to focus on.

The gastrocnemius and soleus muscles are in your calves. These muscles help power jumps, runs, and dancing. If you are one of those women who refuse to wear flats, realize that walking in heels is essentially the equivalent to walking on your tiptoes all day long, which forces your calves to be in a constant state of flex. Calf muscles can easily be torn during simple recreational activities like tennis and dance. To avoid injury, gradually warm up these muscles before intense activity and be sure to stretch after you exercise.

The tibialis anterior muscles are located in your shins. They are the opposing muscles to your calves. The function of the shins is to point and flex the feet. Shins are easily aggravated during exercise, creating painful "shin splints." Because this injury is so common, I have devoted a shole section to preventing shin spints below.

Injury Prevention

While weight loss and muscle gain likely top your list of fitness goals, it is essential that we talk about injury prevention. If you injure yourself, that's it; you are out of the game (for a short or long time depending on your injury) and you will fall back into the shape you were in—the same shape that made you realize you needed to move your body and shed some fat in the first place—or more likely into worse shape. The point of exercise is to make your body and mind feel good, to increase your longevity, and to make life that much more worth living. Suffering an injury is like going backward.

Shin Splints

Shin splints are a painful but common injury, often caused by exercising without properly warming up or cooling down. You can avoid shin splints by making sure you always warm up and cool down before and after exercise, wearing the proper athletic shoes for the activity you're engaged in, and gradually increasing your difficulty.

CAUSES OF SHIN SPLINTS

Your Body:

- Weak shin muscles that are suddenly overtrained
- Tight calf muscles or tendons that pull the shins
- Excessively high arches
- Flat feet
- Pronation caused by collapsed arches

Your Gear:

- Shoes that have insufficient shock absorption
- Shoes that lack sufficient stability and motion control
- Shoes that don't support your arches (especially a concern for those with high arches)
- Shoes that are inappropriate for your activity (e.g., don't wear basketball shoes for running)
- Shoes that are old or don't fit properly

Your Environment:

- Exercising on a surface that's too hard
- Exercising on an uneven surface
- Running up or down hills
- Running along banked surfaces, forcing one foot to run at a higher level than the other
- Running in cold weather without first warming up

Your Training:

- Upping your mileage too quickly
- Upping your intensity/speed too quickly
- Running with poor technique
- Doing jumping exercises that shock the legs and splinter the shins
- Running on your toes

As soon as you start feeling shin splints, immediately stop your exercise. The more you run or jump with shin splints, the worse they will become.

TREATMENT FOR SHIN SPLINTS

- *Ice.* Ice is always the first form of defense when you feel that you have overworked a muscle. The reason: ice helps to remove blood and inflammation from the injured area, allowing it to heal more rapidly. If you feel shin splints coming on, ice your shins for twenty minutes.

- *Compression.* Compressing a painful spot is one of our natural reactions for a reason. It activates the healing process. If you get hit in the arm with a baseball, one of your first instincts is to tightly grasp the tender area. Like icing, putting pressure on the injured area helps reduce inflammation. You can apply consistent pressure with a fabric bandage. Or double up your resources by tightly wrapping an ice pack on the injury.
- *Elevation.* Whenever you have an injury you should elevate the injured body part above your heart to minimize blood flow to the area. If you feel shin splints coming on, elevate your shin above heart level while simultaneously icing it and applying compression.
- *Pain Reliever.* Pain relievers that contain ibuprofen do more than minimize pain; they help to reduce inflammation, too.
- *Rest.* Take a week off from the exercise that caused the shin splints and focus on other exercises.

HOW TO AVOID SHIN SPLINTS

Your Body:

- When complementary muscles (like your shins and calves or your back and stomach) are equally strong, your likelihood of injury is decreased. Calf muscles are typically stronger than shin muscles. Strengthen your shins by doing toe raises (as opposed to heel raises, which are for your calf muscles) by pulling your toes up toward your knees. Walking backward or forward on your heels also helps to strengthen the shins.
- After warming up, stretch your calf muscles to minimize their tendency to pull the shins.
- Massage your calf muscles. To get even deeper, use a hard foam roller to roll out the muscle tension.
- Use arch supports or orthotics in your shoes to help support the shape of your soles and the arches in your feet.

Your Gear:

- Wear shoes that have better shock absorption and that help stabilize and control your motion.
- Check that your shoes support your arches. If you can't find any that are sufficient, buy arch supports or orthotics.
- Buy shoes that support your favored activity. Keep in mind that running, aerobic, and walking shoes are all very different, with different support mechanisms to help that specific style of movement.
- Be sure your shoes fit—in the store! You are not supposed to break in shoes.
- Replace your shoes often, every 500 to 750 miles or every six months.

Your Environment/Training:

- Running on soft surfaces is easier on your entire body and will help give your shins, knees, and ankles longevity. Instead of concrete, run on grass, dirt, sand, or designated running tracks.
- If you run on sloped surfaces, like along the side of the street, be sure to switch sides to take some pressure off the upward leg.
- Gradually introduce new elements into your workout, like hills and jumping.
- *Warm up*, especially in cold weather, when your muscles may be colder and need more warming up than in warmer weather.

Stretching

If you want to lose weight long term, you have to stretch. Stretching seemingly (and often actually) elongates your body by retraining your muscles to stand taller as you stack your spine straight, resist slouching, and hold your head higher. It also, and most important, helps with injury prevention. I know, no one wants to talk about preventative measures to avoid potential problems—you feel great right now. But if you twist an ankle, break a leg, or worse, tear a hamstring, because you haven't stretched properly, you will have to pare down your exercise program while you are healing and be more vigilant about ramping it back up once you are injury free.

Look, you can't live long, lean, and healthfully if you tear a muscle right out of the gate. A well-designed fitness program that is intended to keep you stronger and leaner longer gradually increases in intensity so you can ease your body to the next level without causing injury.

But don't just stretch. You have to make sure you are stretching correctly. So, let's get this straight: yes, I want you to stretch, but you shouldn't stretch a cold muscle—ever! Wait until you are slightly warmed up so that your muscles are more malleable, allowing you to stretch more effectively without tempting injury.

Stretching cold muscles can also make your workout less efficient. Static stretching immediately before working out can actually slow you down. Researchers at Jewish General Hospital in Montreal found that after stretching, muscles produce less force. But that

Motivate to Move

One of the biggest complaints of new exercisers who are just getting into the program and establishing a routine is "I don't have the time." You don't have time? I have worked with busy performers whose lives consist of flying from one country to the next, going city to city on tour buses every day, then doing press, autograph signings, sound checks, and rehearsals, and finally performing in front of tens of thousands of screaming fans every night. These people don't have time for family or friends; they don't even have time to make phone calls to stay in touch with people, yet somehow they find both the time and the energy for their regular workouts. They make the time because of the benefits—both physical and mental. When I trained Madonna we worked out probably 330 days each year. In that period she had a legal pad listing her daily responsibilities: meetings, interviews, signings, approving artwork and outfits—but first on her list was always her workout.

doesn't mean you should ditch stretching altogether. Daily stretching *after* exercise can help increase range of motion and athletic ability.

Now let's get that body moving!

Toning Tactics

If you want to slim and not bulk, it's important to understand how to work your muscles and how much weight to use.

Reps and Sets

The theory that the combination of light weight and many repetitions is the way to get toned but not buff is wrong.

I can't tell you how many women have told me, "I don't lift heavy weights because I don't want to get big." Those same women aren't experiencing change for that exact reason. Unfounded fear is holding them back from shaping their Star Quality body. The reason you should do resistance exercises is to fatigue your muscles, breaking them down so that they can build themselves back up even stronger. To fatigue your muscles faster, and therefore see results faster, you need to lift heavy weights fewer times, not the opposite. Why? First, there is the efficiency factor: it just takes too long to get any results when you have to do hundreds of reps to feel anything. Second, oxygen comes into play: instead of fatiguing the muscle and becoming stronger, you are suffocating your muscle, draining it of all its oxygen until finally it gives out and fatigues simply because it has no other choice, which is not helping in the strength department.

The number of reps you should be able to do at a time is 10 to 25, with the last 3 being difficult. After two or three sets, those last 3 reps should end with momentary muscle failure—basically, your muscle loses its ability to function for just a moment. That's how you know you have pushed your muscle to its edge and are effecting change. Work your muscles efficiently; you want them to fatigue because they are working hard, not because they have run out of oxygen.

More Than for Your Skinny Jeans

Don't just exercise to fit into your skinny jeans. Extend your life by staying in shape.

If Americans would improve their diets, be more physically active, keep their weight under control, and not smoke, 90 percent of diabetes, 80 percent of heart disease, and 60 percent of all cancers could be prevented. In fact, just dropping 10 percent of your weight can significantly reduce your risk of several major diseases. And you are almost guaranteed to be happier! In fact, studies have shown that overweight women who start and stick with an exercise and diet program are almost immediately happier and more energetic.

The benefits of taking off the pounds are phenomenal.

- Burning off five to ten pounds will cut your chances of developing type-2 diabetes in half, help prevent osteoarthritis by reducing the load on your knees (for every pound you lose, there is a four-pound reduction on the load bearing down on your knees), and minimize your risk of heart disease (for every percent of weight you drop, you reduce your chance of heart disease by 1 to 2 percent).

- Burning off ten to twenty pounds will lower your breast cancer risk by 34 to 53 percent, according to a study conducted at the University of Toronto. Other studies have shown that women who regularly walk, bike, or do any other moderate movement activity reduce their risk by 20 percent. It will also slash your blood pressure. One study showed that people who lost fifteen pounds reduced their risk of developing hypertension by 28 percent.

- Burning off twenty to thirty pounds will cut your risk of all cancers, make your sex life more satisfying, and help you get a better night's sleep—approximately half of all sleep apnea cases (when you stop breathing, forcing you to wake up several times during the night) are caused by excess weight.

If you are at a healthy weight, your job is to tone your muscles and maintain your weight. You don't want to let yourself get too thin! Anorexia is not a joke. It is a sickness that can do serious long-term damage to your body and life. I have seen it. It isn't a pretty way to live.

Maintaining a healthy weight, on the other hand, has some serious benefits. Studies show that yo-yo dieters have a 40 percent lower immune system than women who are able to maintain a healthy weight for more than five years. Yup, roller-coaster dieting increases your chances of getting colds, herpes, and other viral infections, and even cancer. Your risk for high blood pressure, high cholesterol, and gallbladder disease also dramatically increases.

ON-THE-GO EXERCISE

Short on time? Since *Star Quality* uses glitz and glam to create a complete fitness routine, when you don't have the time to do a full workout, you can still do something. Take one or two exercises from each category to create your own on-the-go workout. You can also choose to do a quick transitional workout—meaning that you will work out one muscle group to fatigue, then switch to an adjacent muscle group. For example, try push-ups followed by tricep dips. Just don't make this skimping trick a habit. It is an exception, not the rule.

6

Star Quality Food

Food is fuel. That's how you have to view it. Yes, you can enjoy your meals. You can dine out. You can savor every bite. But you have to stop looking at food as a source of comfort and view it as the fuel that allows you to exercise, play with your kids, perform at the office—live your life. Food's function, at its most basic, is to provide energy for the body.

Food provides the nutrients to support your fitness and your life. If you don't get enough food, if you don't consume enough healthy calories, you won't have enough energy to do a good workout and you will pass out. It's really that simple. You don't want to be skinny or fragile; you want to be lean and tough. You get that way by eating nutritiously.

The Celebrity Skinny

So how is it that celebrities stay so slim? They don't just exercise; they eat right. They think before they shovel fried chicken into their mouths (or they pay someone like a chef or a nutritionist to think for them). That doesn't mean that they stay away from the greasy stuff altogether. Moderation is key.

If you want to know the truth, celebs have it the worst when it comes to being surrounded by fatty, sugary, high-carb, high-calorie, greasy foods. Maybe not at home, but on the movie or TV set (sometimes for upward of twelve hours each day) they have what the entertainment industry calls "craft services." Craft services is the catering company that sets up camp on the set, supplying sustenance to the actors and the crew. The problem with craft services is that they are there to serve everyone, and not everyone is watching his or her weight. While there are the requisite crudités (a fancy word for cut, cold, uncooked vegetables), much of the food available—particularly the snacks served between meals—consists of high-fat, high-calorie, high-sugar, high-salt, energy-spiking nibbles that quickly add up.

So celebs have to think before they gorge: Is this face-size chocolate chip cookie, with 30 grams of fat, 400 calories, and 50 grams of carbs, worth ruining my diet over? No. But a mini chocolate-covered peppermint patty could do the trick to give me a burst of energy, freshen my breath, satisfy my sweet tooth, and calm my chocolate craving.

It's all about balance and moderation.

Here are some Star Quality nutritional tips to get you through the day.

- Eat a small meal and or a snack five to six times a day.
- Include protein with every meal.
- Choose carbohydrates in the form of fruits and vegetables with every meal.
- Eat monounsaturated and polyunsaturated fats with each meal. Limit saturated fats from animal products. Avoid trans fats (hydrogenated oils).
- Don't drink your calories. Avoid sodas, sports drinks, alcohol, and mixers. Keep your system hydrated with water.

Naomi Watts Fuels Up with Fruit

Naomi loves fruit. So I created a fruit salad that would give her sustained energy all day—watermelon, cantaloupe, apples, strawberries, and oranges. It is filled with vitamins and minerals to help keep her immune system strong, her body healthy, and her energy high. It is also filled with flavor!

- Eat organic foods whenever possible.

- Supplement your diet with fish oil (omega-3), vitamin C, B complex, an antioxidant compound, flaxseeds or flaxseed oil, calcium, magnesium, and iron.

- Listen to your body.

- Aim for a combination of 30 percent carbohydrates, 40 percent protein, and 30 percent fats.

This isn't a diet plan. Your focus should not be on restrictions. This is a nutritional plan that will lay out the most effective way to eat in order to best support your life's activities and sustain your energy and blood-sugar level throughout the day. I am not here to tell you to starve or deny yourself your favorite things. Life is about balance.

I won't ask you to count your calories, but I will ask that you keep track of what and how much you put into your mouth (this includes grazing—one cookie here, four fries there, a chip or two . . .). When calories consumed outnumber calories burned, you are sure to bulge. When it comes down to it, that is why you are fat—you eat too much and you don't burn off enough.

When to Fuel

Eat after your workout. But if you work out first thing in the morning, it is important to break your fast (the ten or so hours since you ate the night before) by having a light carbohydrate, like a banana or 8 ounces of orange juice, before your workout. Breakfast helps wake up your body and gets it moving. About twenty minutes after you complete your workout, you should eat a real meal, with an emphasis on proteins.

For evening exercisers, the same rule applies. You don't want to work out on a completely empty stomach, but you also don't want to eat a hearty meal before hopping on your bike or slipping on your

Drink Coffee!

If you prefer to exercise early in the morning after a cup of coffee, doing so actually might help ease the pain of a strenuous workout. Recent studies suggest that drinking two cups of coffee before you exercise may reduce postexercise muscle pain by as much as 50 percent!

running shoes. Why? Your food needs to digest, a process that requires extra blood and enzymes to be delivered to your stomach in order to start breaking down the food. If you work out right after eating a full-scale meal, there is a good chance your stomach will cramp up as the muscles that you are exercising wrestle with your stomach for the blood that is needed to both digest your food and power your body to move. Eat something healthy and small two hours before you work out at night. After you exercise you can have your meal, but make sure it isn't too heavy. Contrary to popular belief and practice, your last meal of the day should be your lightest.

More important than when you eat is what you eat and how much. Making good choices and practicing portion control are key when it comes to eating a healthy diet.

Americans have adopted a hoarding mentality that makes us want to eat as much as we can at every meal. We expect to sit down in front of big plates covered in hearty servings of food. Then we eat and eat and eat until we have to unbutton our pants for fear of bursting. You know you do it, too. We care less about quality and more about quantity. Why do you think so many buffet-style, all-you-can-eat restaurants thrive? Because we don't care how fresh the vegetables are or if the meat is organic, all we care about is getting "our money's worth."

Ever wonder why the French and the Italians don't seem to pack on the pounds like we do despite the fact that they dine on pasta, bread, cheese, chocolate, and wine? Because they enjoy small servings of their flavor-filled foods. They don't have the "This is so good, I need to eat all of it" mentality that we do. Instead, they savor a few bites and look forward to enjoying the food again in the future. Then after dinner they socialize by walking. It is a very healthy and balanced approach to life and fitness.

Water

Let's talk about the one type of fuel that is even more important than food—water. You can live without food for weeks, but you could only survive without water for three or four days before you would die.

Water makes up a large percentage of the body—approximately 62 percent of average adult men, 51 percent of average adult women, 71 percent of adult male runners, 70 percent of adult female gymnasts, and only about 48 percent of obese men and women combined. Water is present in every single cell in your body, from your skin to your tendons. Water is essential in the disposal of toxins from your body. It maintains your body's temperature, ensuring that you don't overheat (one of the reasons you sweat is to release heat) or freeze. Water acts as a cushion for your organs so that they don't bang into one another and rupture while you go about your daily business. It helps your digestive system efficiently process your food by pulling out essential nutrients, breaking food down, and separating out the waste. Your muscles depend on water to keep them lubricated and avoid cramping. Water is essential for energy. Think about it this way: the more water you drink, the more energy you have, the harder you can work out, the more calories you can burn, the more weight you can lose faster!

How do you know if you really are thirsty? Well, if you think you're thirsty, you are already beyond thirsty and well into dehydration. Your body doesn't alert you that there is a water deficiency until there is one. To avoid dehydration, drink water all the time! The thing about dehydration is that sometimes it's hard to read. You may think you're hungry, so you reach for a calorie-loaded snack, when really your body is craving water (which could be why you go for watermelon or another high-water content food). If you feel hungry, first drink a glass of water. Let it sit for a few minutes, allowing it to digest a little. Then decide if you are actually hungry or if it was water your body was calling out for.

It's a good idea to drink a glass of water before every meal. Water is a great filler, taking up space in your stomach that you could otherwise have filled unnecessarily with food. Since not eating until we feel like bursting is such a challenge for so many Americans, this is a quick, easy, and free way to help you battle the bulge.

You can lose a quart of water during one workout. You can lose a pint of water just through your feet during the course of a day! There is a reason you should drink at least eight glasses of water every day (more than eight glasses for those of you who are engaging in strenuous activity). You naturally lose water all day without even knowing it. With each exhale a small amount of water escapes your system (think about that steam you leave on glass when you breathe on it). It slowly and discreetly drips out of your pores.

Remember that there are literally hundreds of thousands of pores covering the surface of the body, each of which drips sweat. When you exercise outside, with the fresh air and wind pushing against your body, you may appear to sweat less than when you work out in a gym. That doesn't mean the sweat is dripping out any slower. It's just disappearing into the air before you get a chance to notice it. But more than eliminating water, sweat secretes toxins that your body needs to get rid of in order to maintain your healthy system. Yet another reason for a good hard sweat session—detoxification!

Sweating is one of the main contributors to water loss. But a hard workout triggers it in other ways, too—working out makes you breathe more deeply and rapidly, increasing the amount of water loss.

The bottom line is, hydrate!

To avoid dehydration, it is important to drink at least one glass of water an hour before you begin your workout. This way you give your body the chance to digest the water and avoid that sloshing feeling in your stomach. Then, thirty minutes before you begin your workout, drink another glass of water. Avoid drinking too much more between this time and the time you actually start to move your body—again, to allow the water time to begin to digest. Throughout your workout, have a few gulps of water every twenty minutes to replenish natural water loss. Once you have completed your workout, drink another two glasses of water to rehydrate.

Here's the lowdown on what's good to drink and what should be avoided.

Good: Water, tea (green, black, or white), red wine (in moderation—and not for hydrating)

Decent: Black coffee, diet soda (in moderation), 100 percent juice fruit juices, white wine, light beer, smoothies (in moderation—smoothies are high in calories, sugars, and carbs)

Bad: 10 percent juice fruit juices (the other 90 percent is sugar), hard alcohol, powdered juices, soda, wine coolers

How to Work a Diet into Your Life without Going Crazy

Diets are hard to keep up with. No one wants to feel restricted or be told that you can't have what you most want—like a cookie or a bag of chips. Then there are the diets that allow you to eat anything you want, but you can eat only 1,200 calories a day. One cookie might have 300 calories. So then what? You try to do a calorie breakdown that allows you to splurge in a controlled manner. You measure and weigh portions, you keep a tally of calories and fat consumed, you obsess about your meals, on what you can and cannot have, and you finally lose count, get frustrated, feel starved, and give up!

And that is the biggest problem with diets. They don't work well with your lifestyle. They force you to fixate on food because you are always thinking about it.

You shouldn't feel restricted. You shouldn't feel as if you are counting calories. The only way to work a diet into your life is to not allow it to make you crazy, but to actually feel good about it. The only way to really feel good about your diet is to look at food and its purpose differently.

Look at each meal and think about what benefits it will give you. Does it have enough protein to help you build muscle? Does it have enough carbohydrates to give you sustained energy without throwing you on a roller coaster of ups and downs? Eating with intention helps you avoid scarfing down food without even acknowledging the taste.

Some people really enjoy the concept, experience, and luxury of truly dining, on meals that are drawn out and feature flavor- and fat-filled morsels that make their taste buds sparkle like Christmas-tree lights. You can still have that experience. You can savor your food. But you don't need to have a full-fat experience at every meal. I am not as concerned with special occasions as I am with your day-to-day diet. What did you eat for breakfast? What was your midmorning snack? What about lunch? Did you have a healthy afternoon snack? And dinner? I will show you how your food can work for you. It is really very simple.

The breakdown of your meals should be:

Carb and protein for breakfast

Protein-rich 120-calorie midmorning snack

Balanced lunch of proteins and vegetables

Protein-rich 120-calorie afternoon snack

Balanced dinner of protein and vegetables

Does that sound like a lot of food? For some of you it may be. Eating those two extra snacks may make you feel you're overdoing it. But you aren't. The fact is that keeping your metabolism pumping will keep you burning calories, helping to make the fat fall off. Just choose snacks low in fat and calories but high in protein. Then try to minimize the size of your main meals, too, in order to balance your diet and make it relatively consistent all day long.

I don't swear by the Food Guidance System (also known as the food pyramid), but I think it is a good guide and can help you understand food choices and balance. The food pyramid is that triangle you might notice on some packaged foods like breads and cereals. You might also notice that the pyramid doesn't look the same as it used to. That's because it was recently updated to address our current health issues. The pyramid has been pushed over onto its side, and along the slope is a staircase with a person running up, highlighting the importance of exercise as part of a healthy lifestyle. The triangle is filled with six colored strips, each a different width, corresponding to fruits and vegetables, grains, proteins, fats, and sugars and how much of each you should consume each day. There are also dietary guidelines to remind you of how to eat healthfully, such as:

Balance and variety are essential.

Eat plenty of fruits, vegetables, and grains.

Keep fat and sugar to a minimum.

Just remember that the Food Guidance System offers *guidance*. Take what makes sense to you and your specific needs. Don't follow it to the letter if it doesn't work with your body. The only guidance you have to follow to the letter is mine. Hey, that's what you're paying me for.

Chances are that even with the Food Guidance System, you're still confused about what to eat. Which carbs are considered "good" and which "bad"? What fats should you avoid and what fats should you be sure to eat every day? What types of sugars are good for you and what types are not? Here's where the hand-holding comes in—don't get used to it. Following is a discussion about what to eat and what not to eat.

Up the Ante

Time Your Meals

Research suggests that waiting to eat until after your workout can motivate your body to tap into your fat stores and burn more calories while exercising. On the other hand, if you're feeling famished, eat! Hunger to the point of weakness will slow you down and make you burn less calories.

Protein

I am a big believer in protein. It helps your body heal after exercise. It helps build muscle, which naturally increases your calorie burn. And it provides sustained energy. Eating protein or drinking a protein shake after a workout will also dramatically minimize muscle soreness the next day. But that doesn't mean you should go overboard and eat only protein. Remember that you have to keep your diet balanced.

Focus on baked, broiled, or grilled fish and lean meats like chicken, turkey, ostrich, and buffalo and leaner cuts of red meats, such as round eye, top round, bottom round, round tip, top loin, top sirloin, ham, tenderloin, and center loin. Vegetarians need to be extra careful to get enough protein. Good sources of nonanimal proteins include beans (kidney beans, pinto beans, chickpeas), tofu, tempeh, and nuts (almonds, walnuts, pine nuts, cashews, pecans).

When it comes to protein, how you prepare it is essential for maintaining its healthy benefits. As soon as you drop a piece of chicken into the fryer or slather that steak with butter, you are adding fat to what otherwise can be a healthy food. Do not fry your food! That crunch is pure fat! Even stir-frying can be unhealthy. Unless you stir-fry in broth or fat-free sauces, or use minimal oil, you are saturating your meal in, yes, fat. Say good-bye to greasy bacon (unless it is low-fat bacon cooked with cooking spray), chicken wings, fried fish fillets, even french fries—if not for your butt, then for your heart. That excess oil clogs arteries.

More than a steady-burning fuel, providing long-term energy that helps build muscle mass, protein is high in iron. Much of the body's iron is stored in the blood, leaving you in short supply during your menstrual cycle. In order to avoid iron deficiency, you should up your protein intake after your cycle as well as during pregnancy. Iron-rich vegetarian options include spinach, beans, raisins, prunes, lima beans, navy beans, black beans, peas, broccoli, Swiss chard, asparagus, parsley, watercress, and Brussels sprouts, as well as iron-fortified pastas, bread, cereals, and other whole grains.

Here's where it gets tricky: just because you are eating your protein and iron doesn't mean

---

Essential Elements

Iron and Exercise

Approximately 90 percent of women aren't getting enough iron. Because much of it is stored in red blood cells, and you lose a lot of blood each month during your cycle, women require twice as much iron as men do—18 milligrams each day. You will know that your iron stores are low when you are excessively tired, your mind is fuzzy, and you feel as if you don't have the energy to exercise (of course, these are symptoms of several other things, too, but don't dismiss the possibility that it is an iron deficiency as opposed to lack of sleep). The reason for the excessive exhaustion is that iron assists in the transportation of oxygen from your red blood cells to your muscles and your brain. Not sure if you are getting enough natural iron in your diet? Routine blood work at your doctor's office will tell you your iron level. If it is too low, your doctor may prescribe a supplement.

your body is benefiting. To efficiently absorb iron, you have to be sure you are consuming foods that are high in vitamin C, because one of vitamin C's many purposes is to assist in the absorption of iron. So why is this so important that I am dedicating a paragraph to it? Because when you are iron deficient, you can become anemic. Anemics suffer from irritability, dizziness, headaches, and exhaustion—none of which helps my cause, which is to get you to work out. Let's face it, you are less likely to stick to your fitness routine if you are constantly walking around feeling as if you are going to faint.

Before you open your fridge and grab a chicken leg or a sausage link, become familiar with the good, the decent, and the bad protein options. What determines the quality of a protein is its fat content. With the exception of a few of the fatty fishes that are very high in omega-3 fatty acids such as salmon, mackerel, lake trout, herring, sardines, and albacore tuna, high-quality proteins are low in fat.

Following are protein sources and the categories they belong to.

Good

- *Fish/seafood*: abalone, albacore tuna, anchovies, bass, calamari, clams, cod, crab, crawfish, flounder, grouper, halibut, herring, lake trout, lobster, mackerel, mahimahi, mussels, oysters, salmon, sardines, scallops, shark, shrimp, snapper, swordfish
- *Poultry*: chicken (white meat, skinless), eggs, ground turkey (extra lean), turkey breast (skinless)
- *Meat*: beef (filet mignon, extra lean ground beef), buffalo, pork (ham, Canadian bacon), venison
- *Legumes*: black beans, chickpeas, kidney beans, lima beans, navy beans, pinto beans, soybeans (edamame), tofu
- *Dairy*: cheeses (less than 2 percent fat), Egg Beaters, egg whites, milk (fat-free), yogurt (low-fat, low-sugar, plain)

Decent

- *Poultry*: chicken (white meat with skin), turkey (white meat with skin, turkey bacon, 85 to 90 percent lean ground turkey)
- *Meat*: beef (85 to 90 percent lean ground beef, bottom round,

flank steak, roast beef, round eye, round tip, stews, top loin, top round, top sirloin), duck, pork chops

- *Dairy*: cottage cheese (1 to 2 percent fat), milk (1 to 2 percent fat), whole eggs, yogurt (whole milk, low-fat/low-sugar frozen)

Bad

- *Meat*: beef (fatty cuts like New York strip, T-bone, chuck, and ground beef with more than 15 percent fat), foie gras, hot dogs, liver, pâté, pepperoni, pork (bacon, sausage), salami
- *Dairy*: hard cheeses, milk (whole, cream)

Fruits and Vegetables

You have to eat more fruits and vegetables. With few exceptions, the average American does not consume even close to the daily suggested amount of fruits and vegetables. No, that piece of parsley garnishing your pork chops or the lettuce leaf adding a dash of green to your lamb loin doesn't count. The goal is to eat five servings of a variety of fruits and vegetables every day. I am talking about a plate covered in colors—red bell peppers, green asparagus, yellow onions, red tomatoes, green spinach, and white cauliflower. Make fruit salads with bananas, blueberries, raspberries, grapes, melon, and grapefruit. The more colors, the more essential vitamins and nutrients—and the deeply colored vegetables can actually minimize your risk of cardiovascular disease and certain cancers. Your fruits and veggies are most efficient at delivering the nutrients your body needs when they are fresh. Frozen is okay, too. Only opt for canned if fresh or frozen is not available. Canned fruits and vegetables are often very high in sodium and can be depleted of many nutrients.

Fruits and vegetables are the first fast food! Grab an apple, a banana, or an orange, cut up carrots, celery sticks, or radishes, and you have a healthy, fast, and convenient snack. For a completely balanced snack, combine dried berries and almonds in a plastic bag and stash it in your purse for instant gratification.

Not only will upping your intake of fruits and vegetables keep your waist slim, it will help you maintain good health—fruits and vegetables have been proven to aid in the prevention of heart disease and cancers. They are brimming with essential nutrients that your body needs and you should learn to want.

Carbohydrates

Not all carbohydrates are bad. Those no-carb diets that millions of people swore by in recent years are not necessarily the answer to weight loss. In fact, they can do more harm than good. I know women who thought that eating three cheeseburgers without the bun for lunch was healthy. That is over 90 grams of fat in one meal—not good! Balance is key.

Stop banning all carbs from your pantry. You need whole grains, rice, and certain breads and pasta to fuel you. But again, you have to strike a balance! Just because I have freed you to eat pasta doesn't mean you can gorge. Be aware of portion sizes. Read the label on a box of pasta. If you aren't sure of what one portion of pasta looks like, look at the preparation directions on the side of the box and prepare exactly one portion (be careful not to confuse serving size and portion size. The recommended preparation amount might be four servings. If that is the case, divide the amount of raw pasta by four and you will be left with the proper serving size for one person—you). Once the pasta is cooked, you will see how big a portion size really is—believe me, it's not much. Those Italian restaurants serving up heaps and piles of noodles are often trying to shove as many as six servings down your throat! Add cheese, and you have just eaten the equivalent in fat and calories of an entire large pizza or a container of ice cream. Just because it fits on the plate doesn't mean it is the amount you should eat. If you feel the need to cover your plate with food, go out and buy smaller plates! Carbs alone are not fattening, but carbs in excess are high in calories and eating too many high-calorie carbs can make you fat.

Keep in mind that I did say "certain breads and pasta" for a reason. There is a difference between "good" carbs and "bad" carbs, "good" breads and pasta and "bad" breads and pasta. They are also differentiated by simple carbs and complex carbs. Simple carbs are bad for you and should be eaten only in moderation. They include white bread, white rice, white flour, and granulated sugar. Complex carbs, including multigrain bread and cereal and wild or brown rice, are filled with healthy fiber, which keeps your digestive system regular. Simple carbs do not contain fiber. They are empty calories and not worth eating.

Good carbs have several things in common.

- *They are high in fiber.* Fiber helps you stay fuller longer, which boosts energy, lowers cholesterol, and minimizes hunger cravings. Fiber also keeps your digestive system pumping, pushing out waste and keeping your system healthy and clean.
- *They have a low glycemic index.* A low glycemic index helps stabilize blood-sugar levels and balance insulin production.
- *They are rich in nutrients.* Nutrient-rich foods filled with vitamins and minerals help fight disease and promote health.
- *They have low-energy density.* With the exception of nuts, low-energy-density foods maintain energy levels and encourage weight loss.
- *They have a high thermic effect.* The thermic effect is the heat-fueled intensity at which metabolism churns and fat burns away.

Now let's break down carbs into good, bad, and decent.

Good

- *Breads*: 10-grain breads (these are the nutty, seedy, grainy, crunchy breads), pumpernickel, rye, sourdough, tortillas (flax-seed, whole-grain)

Little Daily Extras Add Up

You may think that just a handful of peanuts, two pieces of bread with butter before dinner, or a quick afternoon sandwich cookie is an innocent indulgence. Think again! Just two handfuls of peanuts eaten while sitting at a bar are about 420 calories, those two predinner pieces of bread (you know, the kind that is casually dropped off at your table at a restaurant) are about 225 calories, and that afternoon cookie is about 160 calories. Before allowing your hand to thoughtlessly stuff food into your mouth, think! Are those extra calories worth it?

- *Cereals*: bran cereals (with low sugar content), Kashi, oatmeal (slow cooked, not instant)
- *Whole grains*: bran (with low sugar content), buckwheat, kamut, oatmeal (slow cooked, not instant), quinoa, and wheat
- *Pasta/rice*: brown rice
- *Vegetables*: high-fiber fruits and vegetables (not including potatoes), such as beets, sweet potatoes, and yams, as well as whole vegetables such as asparagus, bell peppers, broccoli, Brussels sprouts, carrots, celery, cucumbers, eggplant, field greens, green beans, mushrooms, romaine lettuce, snap peas, spinach, squash, tomatoes
- *Fruit*: apples, blackberries, blueberries, cantaloupe, cherries, grapefruit, grapes, honeydew, kiwifruit, mangoes, oranges, papaya, peaches, plums, pomegranates, raspberries, strawberries, watermelon
- *Legumes*: black beans, chickpeas, kidney beans, lentils, pinto beans, soybeans (edamame)

Decent

- *Breads*: bran or oat muffins, whole wheat bread
- *Cereals*: corn- and rice-based cereals
- *Pasta/rice*: pearled barley, bulgur, egg noodles, pasta (whole wheat or spinach), rice cakes
- *Vegetables*: iceberg lettuce, yellow squash, zucchini
- *Fruit*: dates (dates are loaded with sugar and high in carbs; I call them "nature's candy"), no-sugar-added fruit juices

Bad

- *Breads*: bagels, English muffins, white bread
- *Cereals*: sugar cereals
- *Pasta/rice*: white pasta, white rice

- *Vegetables*: french fries, potatoes
- *Other*: cakes, doughnuts, frozen yogurt (with sugar), fruit candy, ice cream, sugar-sweetened drinks, white flour

Fiber

Fiber is roughage. It is found in the hulls of rice—the part that is pulled off and tossed when white rice is processed. It is also found in vegetables like lettuce, broccoli, and Brussels sprouts. Food that is high in fiber naturally bulks up when digested, so it makes you feel fuller longer. Plus, fiber-rich foods are often low in calories. Because fiber is indigestible plant parts, your body cannot break it down and distribute the calories to places like your butt. Despite its inability to be digested, fiber slowly moves through the digestive system, keeping your blood-sugar levels consistent and preventing a spike. As it moves through and out of your digestive system, fiber pulls other stuck food products out with it, keeping you regular. It maintains a healthy digestive tract and keeps your system flowing smoothly. A healthy intake of fiber is 30 to 35 grams per day. Studies show that the average American is getting only 10 to 12 grams per day. What about you? Do you qualify as average when it comes to fiber intake?

Fat

Before carbohydrates were banned from our lives, fat was blacklisted from our diets. We went through such an antifat phase that even cookie companies were forced to come up with fat-free options. But because we still had the expectation that our foods would taste sweet and slightly "naughty," sugar and carbs were used in excessive amounts, sometimes making one cookie fat free but filled with as many as 350 calories and 55 carbs!

The problem was that these super-sweet, fat-free, high-calorie cookies simply didn't satisfy our cookie cravings like the kind Mama used to make—with fat. In an attempt to satisfy our dessert cravings, we often devoured entire boxes of those carb-loaded cookies in one sitting! Why? Because what we were craving was a little bit of fat. It didn't dawn on us that had we eaten one 50-calorie cookie with 2 grams of fat, we would have been satisfied and wouldn't have needed to gorge ourselves on an entire box of the less-satisfying fat-free alternative.

The same scenario was played out over dinner. Again in an attempt to avoid the F-word, we turned to pasta—lots of it! We would pile hundreds of fat-free noodles onto a plate and call it a diet. The result of mindless carb bingeing? We got fat.

The point is that we have become so afraid of fat and getting fat that we cling to any extreme fad promising to stop the bulge. Thanks (sort of) to those all-fat, no-carb diets, fat is no longer demonized to the extent that it was. But now we are left completely confused about fat and its impact on how healthy we are. And we remain just as overweight as ever.

Let me clarify a few things for you. Not all fat is fattening. In fact, like carbs, there are "good" fats and there are "bad" fats. It's time to learn the difference.

Polyunsaturated, monounsaturated, saturated, and trans fats are the four main forms of fat. Polyunsaturated fat is the healthiest, and trans fat is the unhealthiest. So let's break it down, from best to worst.

Polyunsaturated Fat

Polyunsaturated, or "good," fat is naturally found in some plant oils—sunflower, safflower, soybean, corn, flaxseed, and sesame seed—as well as in coldwater fish, including salmon, striped bass, tuna, halibut, mackerel, trout, herring, and sardines. When left at room temperature, polyunsaturated fat is liquid (it quasi-solidifies when refrigerated). What makes polyunsaturated fats good for you is that they contain essential omega-3 and omega-6 fatty acids, which have a slew of benefits, including the prevention of heart disease, nerve damage, obesity, diabetes, joint pain, skin problems, mood swings, even cancers.

Monounsaturated Fat

Monounsaturated fat, naturally found in plant oils like those made from olives, peanuts, almonds, walnuts, canola seeds, and avocados, is also considered a good fat. Like polyunsaturated fat, monounsaturated fat is generally liquid when at room temperature.

Monounsaturated oil is considered to be the best oil for cooking due to its high oxidation threshold. In other words, monounsaturated oil can be heated to a high temperature and still remain stable instead of turning into a bad hydrogenated oil. Monounsaturated fat is also considered a cholesterol-lowering fat, which can help fight against heart disease and protect you from certain cancers.

Saturated Fat

Saturated fat is bad fat. It's generally easy to spot because it remains solid when left at room temperature (it does the same thing in your body—stays solid and sticky). Present in fatty meats, saturated fat also abounds in butter, ice cream, cheese, and milk. It is also in coconut, palm, and palm kernel oils.

Saturated fat affixes itself to the cells in your stomach, butt, and thighs, as well as clogs your arteries (which causes heart attacks) and makes cholesterol levels skyrocket. Many scientists and health professionals blame saturated fat for this country's obesity problem. Unless you want to get fat and risk your health, avoid it!

Trans Fat

You can't get worse than trans fat, which is the result of bad fat that has gotten worse or even good fat that has gone bad. It is unsaturated fat that has been hydrogenated—turned into solid fat in order to increase the shelf life of food. Trans fats are found in margarine and shortening and are used in many crackers, cookies, chips, doughnuts, and fried foods. The body doesn't know how to digest trans fat because it is unnatural. Trans fat raises low-density lipoproteins, or LDLs (the "bad" cholesterol), and magnifies your chances of getting heart disease.

The truth about fat is that it is all about balance. You want only 20 percent of your daily calories to be from fat, and fat packs a hearty calorie punch. To be healthy, just stick to the good fats.

The following is a breakdown of certain foods and the fat categories they belong to.

Good: Polyunsaturated

- *Oils*: corn oil, flaxseed oil, soybean oil, sunflower oil
- *Vegetables*: avocados, olives
- *Seeds*: pumpkin, sunflower
- *Nuts*: almonds and almond butter, cashews, pecans, soy nuts, walnuts

---

Food News

You Can Eat Dessert and Still Lose Weight!

Just because you're watching your weight doesn't mean you have to skip dessert. Here are a few easy, low-fat, low-calorie, almost-innocent desserts that you can splurge on with a smile.

Crust-Free Fruit Pie

Combine your favorite fruit (try berries, sliced apples, or sliced peaches) with a sprinkle of cinnamon and a tablespoon of crunchy, large-granulated sugar. Place the mixture in an oven-safe bowl and cook it for 10 to 15 minutes at 375°F. Let cool and enjoy!

Low-Cal Cheesecake Pudding

Combine 2 cups skim ricotta cheese with 1½ tablespoons sugar (add ¼ teaspoon cinnamon to add a little spice). Whip them together in a blender until thoroughly combined. If you like, add a few fresh berries to the mix and blend them in, too. Scoop out the sweet cheese and cover it with sliced berries or peaches for a 175-calorie cheesecake pudding.

Good: Monounsaturated

- *Oils*: canola oil, olive oil, peanut oil
- *Nuts*: macadamia nuts (raw), peanuts (and natural peanut butter)

Bad: Saturated

- *Oils*: cocoa butter, coconut oil, palm oil
- *Dairy*: butter, buttermilk, condensed milk, cream cheese, heavy cream, lard, sour cream, whole-fat ice cream, whole milk
- *Meat*: beef fat, pork fat

Bad: Trans Fat

- many cookies and danishes, croissants, doughnuts, fried onion rings, french fries, margarine, vegetable shortening

Overdoing It . . . Occasionally!

Once in a while, if you accidentally, or even intentionally, eat way too much, that's okay. If you eat a few too many bites of cake on your birthday, or your spouse's birthday, or your best friend's birthday; if you indulge in an extra serving of turkey, pie, mashed potatoes, or tamales on one of the many annual holidays; or even if you just can't help but dig into the ice cream carton on a rainy day—it's okay. Just remember that not every day is a holiday. That type of justification is how you get yourself into trouble.

If you splurge, don't freak out. Don't tell yourself you have destroyed your diet. Don't let one setback end your healthy attitude. Everyone caves now and then. The last thing I want you to do is think, "Well, I've already screwed up this healthy day. I may as well go all the way and really ruin it." No! You have not ruined everything. Do not have that doomsday attitude. One carton of ice cream is better than one carton of ice cream, a bag of chips, a pizza, and a cheeseburger. That's called a binge. Think rationally and get back on track. If it makes you feel better, eat a little healthier the next day or work

Many of us naturally pack on two pounds a year. You can prevent the slow slip upward by leaving three bites on your plate during every meal—which equals approximately a hundred calories. Subtracting that many unnecessary calories from your daily count will keep those age-related two pounds away.

out for an extra couple of minutes that week. You have not completely sabotaged your program; you've just thrown a very easily remedied wrench into it. Get back on that healthy wagon and keep pushing forward.

Another way to think about your overeating incident is to figure out what propelled you to overeat in the first place. If it was a holiday or special occasion, fine. But if it was because you were depressed, happy, bored, or anxious, it's time you address that issue. Think about what the cause of the splurge was and come up with an alternative so that next time you find yourself in that same situation you already have a healthier fix in mind. Don't forget the reasons you are working out and eating right. Remember your short-term and long-term goals. Don't lose sight of where you're going and why. Stay strong and know I am right here for you.

A Few Basics to Beware Of

You may think that many of your daily food choices are healthy, or at least innocent. But watch out for some of the lesser known fat-making and energy-taking culprits.

Soda

Try to cut out soda, even diet soda. Diet soda may be free of calories, but it is extremely sweet. Remember that we are trying to retrain your food habits. If you cut sugars and sugar substitutes (like those that sweeten diet soda) out of your diet, your *need* for sweets will be reduced and soon disappear altogether. Continuing to feed your sugar cravings, even with calorie-free sweets, is not helping your new food attitude. Yes, calorie-free sodas can make you crave more sweets later, encouraging you to give in to temptation.

Salt

Minimize your salt intake. Americans oversalt food. We sprinkle it in while cooking, then toss on even more at the table. The purpose of salt is to bring out the natural flavors in healthy ingredients. The problem is that when we oversalt we are actually masking food flavors because we are numbing our tongues. Another effect of too much salt is puffiness. Salt can make you bloated by causing your body to retain too much water, so you appear as though you have gained weight. Some women are more sensitive to salt than others. You can test your taste for salt by going without it for a week. For the first few days, your food may seem bland. But once your taste buds readjust, food's natural flavors will emerge. The most effective way to do this challenge is to avoid restaurants, which are known to oversalt food. Then, after a week, go back to your old salty ways and you will notice a significant difference. You will be convinced that everything you eat is oversalted. That is, until you ask a friend who wasn't on your salt-purging diet to taste your food and she promises it tastes normal. Just be sure to immediately go back to your less salty diet before your tongue again becomes numb and you feel you need that extra salt to flavor your food.

Fruit Juice

The average grocery store fruit juice is just as bad for you as sugary sodas. Why? Look at the label. If your preferred juice is labeled "10 percent juice," that means the other 90 percent is sugar and water. Be sure to buy only 100 percent juice. And even that you should dilute with water to minimize the sticky, calorie-loaded sweetness. Yes, fruit is good for you. But when in the concentrated form of juice minus the healthy fiber, it contains a lot of calories and carbs.

Coffee

If you are unable to function without coffee, join the club of approximately 50 percent of Americans who drink coffee regularly. While coffee is debatably good for you (at least it's not bad for you when consumed in moderation), it is easily tainted by your additions—sugar, milk, cream, chocolate, whipped cream, and so on. A café mocha can have as many as 40 grams of fat and 500 calories! That's more than a meal. If you can't break your coffee habit, fine. Just try to reduce your intake to one or two mugs in the morning only and, if you can't drink it black, skip the cream and sugar and try low-fat milk and a sugar substitute instead.

Condiments

Some of the condiments listed below may be classified in ways you wouldn't expect. But remember that fat content isn't the only factor. Too much salt or sugar can force a seemingly innocent condiment into the "decent" or "bad" list. For example, ketchup and relish are fat free, but they are high in sugar and salt. Pesto is made with fresh herbs, but it is also filled with oil. Soy sauce is fat free and made from soybeans, but its strong flavor is emphasized by a significant amount of salt.

- *Good*: balsamic vinegar, black pepper, cayenne pepper, garlic, ginger, herbs/spices (both fresh and dried), horseradish, hot sauce, hummus, mustard, salad dressing (fat free), salsa
- *Decent*: barbecue sauce, ketchup, light "maple" syrup (most "maple" syrup found in grocery stores is actually a combination of flavored high-fructose corn syrup and water; it's only real maple syrup from maple trees if it is labeled that way), pesto, relish, salad dressing (low fat), salt, soy sauce
- *Poor*: "maple" syrup, mayonnaise, salad dressing (full fat), sugar

Put Your Food to Work

Make your food work for you. Certain foods and eating habits can help you burn fat, build muscle, and maintain your energy levels all day long without causing your blood sugar levels to dip.

Energy-Increasing Foods

Complex carbohydrates are broken down into glycogen and converted into energy. These foods include:

- Fruits
- Vegetables (most green, red, purple, and orange vegetables)
- Whole grains

Muscle Building Foods

Remember this equation: exercise + lean protein = muscle.

The general rule is that you want to consume .8 to .9 grams of protein per pound of body weight. Use this list to help you determine how much protein you need to eat each day. Ideally you should eat only lean protein.

LEAN PROTEIN		
Type	*Serving Size*	*Protein Amount*
Chicken	4 ounces	35 grams
Cottage cheese (low fat)	1 cup	28 grams
Cream cheese (low fat)	1 ounce	4 grams
Egg (white only)	1 large	3 grams
Egg (whole)	1 large	6 grams
Fish	6 ounces	40 grams
Milk (low fat or nonfat)	1 cup	8 grams
Pork (lean)	4 ounces	35 grams
Red meat (lean)	4 ounces	35 grams
Tofu (low fat)	6 ounces	30 grams
Tuna (water packed)	6 ounces	40 grams
Turkey (skinless)	4 ounces	35 grams
Yogurt (low fat)	1 cup	13 grams

Food and Your Moods

Food can help keep your mood pleasant and your mind sharp. Here's how to counteract some negative emotions using nutrition:

ANXIETY

Mood-mending food: Five ounces of lean protein, like sliced chicken breast or grilled fish

Protein helps your brain produce dopamine, norepinephrine, and other neurochemicals that keep you calmly alert.

SLEEPLESSNESS

Mood-mending food: One rice cake or a slice of fat-free, 7-grain bread

Eating a small amount of carbs before bed triggers your body to make the calming neurochemical serotonin. Be sure to avoid fat, which slows down serotonin production, making the carbs less effective.

DEPRESSION

Mood-mending food: Fish, raw or cooked

Studies have shown that regularly eating fish can help minimize depression. Sugars, on the other hand, have the opposite effect, making people even more depressed. Next time you are feeling particularly low, pass on the cookies and ice cream and indulge in a big serving of sashimi (that's sushi without the carb-filled rice).

UNHAPPINESS

Mood-mending food: Chocolate

You were right all along! Chocolate does boost your mood. Anadamine, a naturally occurring chemical in chocolate, triggers your brain to create an all-around good feeling. Just be sure to stick with the purest chocolate bar you can find (that means dark chocolate with at least 75 percent cocoa) to avoid the mood-dampening sugars.

FORGETFULNESS

Mood-mending food: Fruit salad or carrot and bell pepper sticks

Your brain is sensitive to free-radical damage, which hinders your brain's ability to properly utilize oxygen—key to a sharp memory. Amp up your diet with antioxidants to help do away with the rampant free radicals. Choose brightly colored foods like blueberries, pomegranates, strawberries, carrots, and bell peppers to get the most antioxidants out of your food.

STRESS

Mood-mending food: A handful of pumpkin seeds

Stress can sap your body of magnesium, which helps you to healthfully handle stress and keep high blood pressure at bay. Infuse your diet with magnesium with on-the-go options like pumpkin and sesame seeds. Halibut and spinach are also magnesium-rich.

Food and Colds, Flu, and Other Ailments

Food can help your body fight off many common ailments.

FLU

Ailment-alleviating food: Shrimp

Shrimp is high in zinc, a naturally occurring mineral that triggers the body to produce more interleukin-2, a protein that helps the body fight off viruses like the flu.

RUNNY NOSE/SORE THROAT

Ailment-alleviating food: Carrots

The vitamin A that creates the orange color of the carrot also helps the body fend off bacteria by fortifying mucus membranes in the nose and the throat.

UPPER RESPIRATORY INFECTION

Ailment-alleviating food: Avocados

Avocados contain the antioxidant vitamin E, which has been shown to help fight off upper-respiratory infections.

COLDS

Ailment-alleviating food: Guava

The loads of vitamin C stored in guava boost the body's resilience to colds by upping the production of cold-fighting cells.

COLDS/FLU

Ailment-alleviating food: Garlic

Garlic is not only pungent, it also packs a potent ailment-fighting punch with its high concentration of the antimicrobial allicin, which has been proven to help prevent illness.

MIGRAINE HEADACHE

Ailment-alleviating food: Lean protein

Lean proteins like those found in soybeans and chicken breast, as well as riboflavin-rich foods like lima beans, yogurt, spinach, peas, kale, and sunflower seeds, help keep your energy high, and can help stop migraines before they start. Just be sure to avoid processed foods like lunch meat, which can be loaded with nitrates. "Good" fats, like the omega-3 fatty acids found in salmon and flaxseeds or fruit oils such as olive and avocado, are anti-inflammatories, which can minimize the pain of a migraine.

IRRITABLE BOWEL SYNDROME

Ailment-alleviating food: Fiber

You may not know that you have it, but irritable bowel syndrome affects one in five Americans. Symptoms include excessive bloating and gas, constipation, diarrhea, and abdominal pain. A high-soluble-fiber diet helps minimize the symptoms. Opt for oatmeal, bananas, and sweet potatoes as opposed to fibers that are hard to digest, like those in most fruits and whole grains.

Start a Food Journal

Face the facts with a food journal. You will be shocked to find out how many little bites, thoughtless nibbles, and quick samples you actually eat each day. Remember that each forkful adds up. Yeah, it's easy to tell yourself that that forkful of your child's macaroni and cheese, that sample-size muffin at the coffee shop, that "just one bite" of cake, doesn't count. Just wait until you have to write each and every one of those extras down and suddenly you will find yourself avoiding them.

This is what your food journal should consist of:

- A daily report of everything you put in your mouth—each bite, every sip, even the piece of hard candy you suck on to avoid eating cake.

- Then, for every guilt-inducing binge, write down the cause (ran into ex), the behavior (ate an entire cake), and the consequence (felt happy at first, then sick, fat, and angry).

- Finally, decide on a new behavior for your most common cause—like window-shopping or going for a run (I promise you it is a lot more pleasing and cleansing than it seems on paper).

Star Quality Meals and Recipes

In this chapter you will find several breakfast, snack, lunch, and dinner options. Because this book is about accessorizing the basics, mix and match to your liking and to keep it interesting!

Breakfast

Organic Yogurt and Fresh Fruit   SERVES 1

1 cup organic vanilla yogurt
½ cup fresh raspberries

½ cup sliced fresh bananas
½ cup fresh blueberries

Place the yogurt in a bowl, top with the fresh fruit, and enjoy. Since you will be using only a small amount of banana, set the rest aside for an afternoon snack.

This is a simple protein- and antioxidant-packed breakfast.

Breakfast Burrito   SERVES 1

Olive oil spray
2 slices low-fat turkey bacon
1 baking or 3 red potatoes, grated
2 tablespoons coconut oil

1 egg, lightly beaten
1 whole wheat flour tortilla
¼ cup fat-free cheese (your preference)

Spray a skillet with olive oil spray and cook the turkey bacon over medium-high heat until it begins to brown. Add the potatoes and coconut oil and cook until the bacon and potatoes are slightly crispy (about 5 minutes). Remove them from the heat to a plate and set aside. Add the egg to the skillet and cook over low heat. Do not stir the egg; instead, allow it to slowly cook and set. Once the egg is set, flip it and cook the other side through.

Lay the tortilla on a plate. Place the egg on the tortilla, add the potato hash, and sprinkle the cheese on top. Roll the tortilla into a burrito and enjoy.

Power Protein Breakfast   SERVES 1

2 eggs
½ pound lean ground beef

Cooking spray
Salt and pepper

Prepare the eggs any way you like and set aside.

Shape the beef into a patty. Spray a skillet with cooking spray and cook the patty to your desired doneness (11 to 18 minutes, depending on the patty's thickness, temperature of the skillet, and your preference).

Add salt and pepper to taste, or to really kick it up a notch, try Worcestershire sauce (my favorite!).

On a plate, stack the eggs onto the patty and enjoy!

Almond Butter and Apple Smoothie   SERVES 1

1½ cups apple juice
½ cup peeled and sliced apple
1 tablespoon almond butter

¼ cup milk (1 percent, 2 percent, or soy)
2 ice cubes

Place all the ingredients in a blender and combine until smooth. Pour into a glass and enjoy.

Add or subtract ice depending on the desired thickness.

Cottage Cheese with Strawberries and Wheat Germ
SERVES 1

¾ cup low-fat cottage cheese
½ cup sliced strawberries

1 tablespoon wheat germ

Place the cottage cheese in a bowl, top with the strawberries and wheat germ, and enjoy.

Egg Whites with Spinach   SERVES 1

½ tablespoon olive oil
½ cup chopped spinach
3 egg whites or ¾ cup liquid
    egg whites

Salt and pepper
1 teaspoon freshly grated Parmesan
    cheese

In a small nonstick sauté pan, heat the olive oil over medium heat. Add the spinach and sauté for 1 minute, or until wilted. Add the egg whites and scramble; season with salt and pepper.

Place the eggs on a plate, sprinkle with the Parmesan cheese, and enjoy.

Tip: I keep liquid egg whites on hand; they are easy to work with and reduce the waste of unwanted yolks. Look for these next to the eggs in your local health food store.

Protein Smoothie   SERVES 1

1 banana
1 scoop protein powder

2 cups low-fat milk

Place all the ingredients in a blender and combine until smooth. Enjoy.

Tip: When choosing a protein powder, opt for one that has no added sugar—it can be soy, rice, whey, or vegetable based.

Egg-White Omelet with Veggies   SERVES 1

½ tablespoon olive oil
⅛ cup diced red bell pepper
¼ cup broccoli, small florets

3 egg whites or ¾ cup liquid egg whites
Salt and pepper
1 tablespoon chopped fresh mozzarella

In a small nonstick sauté pan, heat the olive oil over medium heat. Add the bell pepper and broccoli and sauté for 1 minute, stirring constantly. Add the egg whites and, using a heat-resistant spatula, move the eggs to the center of the pan, allowing them to spill back out to the edges and cook until the eggs are set (about 3 minutes).

Sprinkle with salt and pepper, then add the fresh mozzarella. Fold the eggs in half over the cheese and cook for 30 seconds on each side. Place the folded omelet on a plate. Enjoy!

Midmorning Snack

Apple and Almond Butter

1 small apple

1 tablespoon almond butter

Slice the apple into wedges and dip in the almond butter. Enjoy.

Pumpkin Seeds and Dried Cherries

½ cup pumpkin seeds, roasted

¼ cup dried cherries

Mix together and enjoy.

Cottage Cheese and Cucumbers

½ cup low-fat cottage cheese

2 3 × ½-inch cucumber sticks

Spread a small amount of cottage cheese on the cucumber sticks. Enjoy.

Dried Figs and Almonds

3 figs

¼ cup raw almonds

Mix together and enjoy.

Banana with Almond Butter

½ banana   1 tablespoon almond butter

Dip the banana in the almond butter or spread the almond butter on the banana. Either way, this is a treat.

Hard-Boiled Egg and Vegetable Sticks

1 hard-boiled egg   4 3 × ½-inch cucumber sticks
Salt and pepper

Enjoy with a sprinkle of salt and pepper.

Tip: This is a great snack because it can be prepared ahead of time and taken on the go. Eggs can be boiled several at a time and are great to have on hand for a quick protein fix.

Dried Cranberries and Cashews

¼ cup raw cashews   ¼ cup dried cranberries

Mix together and enjoy.

Almond/Sunflower Butter and Fresh Fruit Sandwich

2 tablespoons almond or sunflower butter   4 large strawberries, thinly sliced
1 slice whole wheat bread

Spread the butter on the whole wheat bread and layer the strawberries on top.

Eat like an open-faced sandwich.

Lunch

Grilled Chicken Breast with Green Beans and Snap Peas
SERVES 1

1 5-ounce skinless, boneless chicken breast   ½ teaspoon minced garlic
1 tablespoon olive oil   Salt and pepper
Juice of ½ fresh lemon   3 ounces green beans
1 teaspoon chopped chives   10 snap peas

Marinate the chicken for at least 30 minutes with ½ tablespoon of the olive oil, the lemon juice, chives, garlic, and a pinch of salt and pepper.

Preheat the grill to 375°F and cook the chicken until the internal temperature is 165°F, as indicated by a meat thermometer inserted into the thickest part of the chicken (about 10 minutes per side).

While the chicken grills, place the green beans, snap peas, and half an ounce of water in a small sauté pan, cover, and steam over medium heat; the water should evaporate in 1 to 2 minutes. Add the remaining ½ tablespoon of olive oil and lightly season with salt and pepper. Sauté for 1 minute.

Plate the chicken and vegetables and enjoy.

Romaine Sandwich   SERVES 1

2 leaves romaine lettuce
4 to 6 slices turkey breast
1 medium tomato, sliced
1 slice low-fat Cheddar cheese

Mustard (optional)
Low-fat mayonnaise (optional)
Salt and pepper

Trim the lettuce leaves (top and bottom) to remove any tough or wilted areas.

If you like, spread mustard and/or low-fat mayonnaise on the leaves. Place the turkey, tomato slices, and cheese on one leaf. Top with the other leaf and eat as you would a sandwich.

Spartan Tuna   SERVES 1

1 can tuna in spring water, drained
1 stalk celery, thinly sliced
¼ cup Dijon mustard

1 leaf romaine lettuce, 1 slice whole wheat bread, or 1 whole wheat tortilla

In a bowl, combine the tuna, celery, and mustard. Blend the ingredients with an electric hand blender until thoroughly combined and chopped.

Serve on romaine lettuce, whole wheat bread, or a whole wheat tortilla as an open-faced sandwich.

Tuscan Salad with Parmesan-Encrusted Salmon   SERVES 1

4 ounces salmon
1 tablespoon extra-virgin olive oil
Salt and pepper
1 tablespoon freshly grated Parmesan
    cheese
3 cups mixed greens
2 tablespoons sliced sun-dried tomatoes

4 calamata olives, pitted and halved
1 tablespoon diced red onion
½ tablespoon fresh oregano
1 teaspoon minced garlic
⅛ cup chopped cucumber
Juice of ½ fresh lemon

Preheat the oven to 375°F.

Place the salmon in an oven-safe pan and lightly drizzle with the olive oil; season with a pinch of salt and pepper and top with the Parmesan cheese.

Bake the salmon for 3 to 5 minutes, depending on the desired doneness.

In a bowl, toss all the remaining ingredients until well combined.

Place the greens on a plate, top with the salmon, and enjoy.

Beet, Goat Cheese, and Marinated Tomato Salad with Toasted Pine Nuts   SERVES 1

1 cup ½-inch beets, chopped into
    cubes
1 tablespoon olive oil, plus more
    for the beets
Salt and pepper
1 cup plum tomatoes, chopped
    into 1-inch cubes

2 tablespoons fresh basil chiffonade
½ tablespoon balsamic vinegar
1 teaspoon fresh minced garlic
6 ounces mixed greens
2 teaspoons pine nuts, toasted
1 tablespoon goat cheese

Preheat the oven to 350°F.

If you are using fresh beets, wash them well. If you are using canned beets, use organic if possible. Lightly drizzle the beets with olive oil and season with a pinch of salt and pepper. Place them in an oven-safe pan with a lid or wrap with foil.

Bake the beets for 40 minutes, or until fork tender. Depending on the size of the beets they could take more or less time to bake.

In a medium bowl, toss the plum tomatoes with 1 tablespoon of the basil, ½ tablespoon of the olive oil, the balsamic vinegar, garlic, and a pinch of salt and pepper. Set aside.

In another medium bowl, toss the mixed greens, beets, pine nuts, and remaining basil and olive oil and season with salt and pepper. Add the marinated tomatoes and lightly toss one more time, being careful not to overmix. You do not want to break up the tomatoes.

Place on a plate, sprinkle with the goat cheese, and enjoy.

Kale Salad with Goji Berries, Pine Nuts, and Balsamic Chicken   SERVES 1

1 6-ounce skinless, boneless
   chicken breast
1 1/2 tablespoons extra-virgin olive oil
1 tablespoon balsamic vinegar
1/2 teaspoon fresh minced garlic
1 teaspoon dried oregano

Salt and pepper
3 cups chopped kale
2 tablespoons Goji berries
1 tablespoon pine nuts, toasted

Preheat the oven or grill to 375°F.

In a small bowl, marinate the chicken breast with 1/2 tablespoon of the olive oil, 1/2 tablespoon of the balsamic vinegar, the garlic, oregano, and a pinch of salt and pepper.

Cook the chicken until the internal temperature is 165°F, as indicated on a meat thermometer inserted into the thickest part of the chicken (about 10 minutes per side). Let cool, then slice and set aside.

Place the kale in a bowl and add the remaining tablespoon of olive oil and the remaining 1/2 tablespoon of vinegar and season with salt. Using your hands, massage the olive oil into the kale to coat the leaves well. Do this for a minute or two, until the kale begins to wilt a bit.

Add the berries and pine nuts and mix. Season with pepper, top with the sliced chicken, and serve.

Tuna Salad Wraps   SERVES 4

For the tuna salad
2 6-ounce cans water-packed
   tuna, drained
1/2 cup nonfat mayonnaise
1/4 cup diced celery
1/4 cup diced sweet onion

For the wraps
4 large whole wheat tortillas
4 leaves lettuce (green leaf, Bibb or
   romaine), shredded
1 large ripe tomato, sliced thin

To make the tuna salad: In a mixing bowl, combine the tuna, mayonnaise, celery, and onion.

To assemble the wraps: Lay out the tortillas on a work surface and divide the tuna mixture among them, spreading it out in the center of each tortilla. Divide the shredded lettuce among the tortillas and top with a slice of tomato. Tightly roll each tortilla into a cylinder, ending with the seam side down.

Cut the wraps in half on the diagonal and serve.

The wraps can be stored in the refrigerator for up to 3 days.

Turkey Burgers   SERVES 4

4 tablespoons fat-free mayonnaise
4 tablespoons barbecue sauce
1 pound lean ground turkey
Salt and pepper

4 whole-grain buns
4 leaves green leaf lettuce
1/2 cup diced tomato

Preheat the grill to medium-high.

In a small bowl, stir together the mayonnaise and barbecue sauce.

Shape the turkey into four patties, each about 1/2-inch thick. Season with salt and pepper and refrigerate until ready to cook.

Grill the burgers on both sides until they are cooked through, about 6 minutes per side. Toast the rolls on the grill until golden brown (about 1 minute).

Top the burgers with the mayonnaise sauce, lettuce, and diced tomatoes and serve them on the toasted rolls.

Roast Beef Sandwiches with Dijon-Horseradish Sauce   SERVES 4

For the Dijon-horseradish sauce
1/4 cup freshly grated horseradish
1 teaspoon Dijon mustard
1/2 cup fat-free sour cream
1/2 teaspoon sugar
Salt

For the sandwiches
8 slices whole wheat bread
3/4 pound roast beef tenderloin,
    sliced
4 leaves lettuce (green leaf, Bibb,
    or romaine), shredded
1 large tomato, sliced thin

To make the Dijon-horseradish sauce: In a small bowl, combine the horseradish, mustard, sour cream, sugar, and salt.

To assemble the sandwiches: Lay out 4 slices of the bread and spread the sour cream mixture on each side. Divide the roast beef among the bread slices. Divide the shredded lettuce among the sandwiches and top with a tomato slice. Cover with the remaining 4 slices of bread.

Cut the sandwiches in half on the diagonal and serve.

Fruit Salad   SERVES 4

2 cups sliced or cubed mixed
   seasonal fruit (apples, oranges,
   berries, or melon)
2 tablespoons orange juice

1 teaspoon chopped fresh mint
2 cups low-fat yogurt or low-fat
   cottage cheese

Mix the fruit in a bowl. Sprinkle with the orange juice and chopped mint, top with the yogurt or cottage cheese, and serve.

Watercress and Endive Salad with Balsamic Vinaigrette   SERVES 4

For the balsamic vinaigrette
1 tablespoon diced shallots
2 tablespoons balsamic vinegar
1/3 cup grapeseed oil
Salt and pepper

For the salad
1 bunch watercress
1 head endive
4 cups shredded rotisserie chicken

To make the balsamic vinaigrette: Place the shallots, balsamic vinegar, and grapeseed oil in a container with a tight-fitting lid. Shake well. Add salt and pepper to taste.

To make the salad: Toss the watercress and endive with the balsamic vinaigrette.

Divide the greens among four plates, top with the chicken, and serve.

Roasted Asparagus Salad   SERVES 4

1½ pounds fresh asparagus
1 tablespoon olive oil
Salt and pepper

2 tablespoons balsamic vinegar
½ cup hummus

Preheat the oven to 350°F.

Prepare the asparagus by cutting off the last inch or so of the woody stalk.

Place the asparagus stalks on a baking sheet, brush them with the olive oil, and sprinkle with salt and pepper. Roast in the oven for 10 minutes, until the stalks begin to get tender on the outside. (Thin asparagus spears will take less time than thick spears.)

Toss with the vinegar and serve with the hummus on the side as a dip.

Quesadillas with Black Beans   SERVES 4

For the salsa
½ cup chopped tomatoes
½ cup chopped red onion
Jalapeño pepper
3 tablespoons diced red bell peppers
1 teaspoon chopped cilantro
1 tablespoon fresh lime juice
Salt and pepper

For the quesadillas
4 large whole wheat tortillas
½ cup low-fat grated Monterey Jack
  cheese
1 15-ounce can black beans, drained
  and rinsed
2 tablespoons chopped cilantro
¾ cup chopped red onion
¾ cup chopped tomato
Low-fat sour cream, for serving

To make the salsa: In a large bowl, combine all the ingredients. (The salsa can be made up to 2 days in advance, covered, and stored in the refrigerator.)

To make the quesadillas: Preheat the oven to 200°F.

Lay out the tortillas on a work surface and arrange the cheese, beans, cilantro, red onion, and tomato on half of each tortilla. Fold over the empty side of the tortillas to cover the filling.

Heat a large nonstick skillet over medium heat. Carefully cook one quesadilla at a time in the skillet until lightly browned on both sides (about 2 minutes per side). Transfer the browned quesadillas to a baking sheet and keep them warm in the oven while cooking the rest.

Slice each quesadilla into four wedges and serve with the salsa and low-fat sour cream.

Hummus and Raw Veggies   SERVES 4

1 8-ounce can garbanzo beans
    (chickpeas), drained and rinsed
1 tablespoon tahini
1 tablespoon lemon juice
1 teaspoon chopped garlic
3 tablespoons olive oil

Salt and pepper
4 whole wheat pitas
4 cups fresh raw vegetables
    (baby carrots, snap peas, radishes,
    celery, broccoli, cherry tomatoes)

Puree the garbanzo beans in a blender or a food processor with the tahini, lemon juice, and garlic. With the machine running, add the olive oil slowly, until the hummus becomes thick and creamy. Add salt and pepper to taste.

Serve with the pita bread and veggies.

Bibb Lettuce Salad with Tuna   SERVES 4

4 cups Bibb lettuce
4 teaspoons diced shallots
2 teaspoons olive oil
1½ teaspoons seasoned rice
    vinegar

2 6-ounce cans water-packed tuna,
    drained
2 hard-boiled eggs, chopped
4 tablespoons Dijon mustard
Salt and pepper

Wash and dry the lettuce and place it in a bowl. Add the shallots, olive oil, and seasoned rice vinegar, and toss until evenly coated. Transfer the salad to four serving plates.

In a separate bowl, combine the tuna, eggs, mustard, and salt.

Top the salad with the tuna, add pepper to taste, and serve.

Hearts of Palm Salad   SERVES 4

1 head butter lettuce
1 14-ounce can hearts of palm,
    drained and cut into 1-inch pieces
1 cup cherry tomatoes
1 medium red onion, sliced

½ cup chopped black olives
1 15-ounce can butter beans, drained
2 cups low-fat cottage cheese
Salt and pepper
Salad dressing

Wash and dry the lettuce, tear the leaves into large pieces, and arrange them on four chilled plates.

Top the lettuce with the hearts of palm, tomatoes, onion, olives, butter beans, and cottage cheese.

Add salt and pepper to taste, drizzle your favorite dressing over the salad, and serve.

Wok Vegetable Sauté SERVES 1

1 tablespoon sesame oil	10 snap peas
½ cup shredded carrots	½ cup chopped baby bok choy
¼ cup chopped celery	3 tablespoons tamari
1 teaspoon minced ginger	1 tablespoon fresh basil chiffonade
1 teaspoon minced garlic	⅛ cup chopped green onions
½ cup sliced mushrooms	½ cup steamed brown rice (optional)

In a large sauté pan, heat the sesame oil over medium heat. Add the carrots and celery and sauté for 1 minute. Add the ginger, garlic, and mushrooms and sauté for 2 minutes, stirring constantly. Add the snap peas and bok choy and sauté for 1 minute, then add the tamari and basil. Garnish with green onion.

Enjoy the vegetables with ½ cup of steamed brown rice if desired.

Balsamic Chicken Salad SERVES 1

1 6-ounce skinless, boneless chicken breast	2 cups romaine lettuce
1 tablespoon olive oil	½ cup sliced cucumber
1 tablespoon balsamic vinegar	1 small tomato, cut into wedges
½ teaspoon fresh minced garlic	⅛ cup chopped green onions, white and green parts
1 teaspoon dried oregano	⅛ cup sliced radicchio
Salt and pepper	

In a small bowl, marinate the chicken breast with ½ tablespoon of the olive oil and ½ tablespoon of the balsamic vinegar, garlic, oregano, and a pinch of salt and pepper for about 20 minutes.

Preheat the oven or the grill to 375°F. Cook the chicken until the internal temperature is 165°F, as indicated by a meat thermometer inserted into the thickest part of the chicken. Set aside.

In a bowl, toss together the remaining ingredients except for the tomato wedges. Season with salt and pepper.

Put the salad on a plate, slice the chicken and place it on top of the salad, arrange the tomatoes around the salad, and enjoy.

Chopped Vegetable Salad with Tuna   SERVES 1

4 ounces water-packed tuna, drained	1/4 cup chopped cucumber
1 teaspoon minced celery	1/4 cup chopped celery
1 tablespoon safflower mayonnaise	1/8 cup chopped green onion
1 teaspoon celery salt	1/4 cup chopped red bell pepper
Pepper	1/4 cup chopped jicama
6 ounces mixed greens	Salad dressing

Place the tuna in a small bowl with the celery, mayonnaise, celery salt, and a pinch of pepper, and mix until incorporated.

In a large bowl, toss the greens and chopped vegetables with your choice of salad dressing. Use a dressing that is olive-oil based and low in saturated fat.

Place the salad on a plate, top with the tuna salad, and serve.

Mediterranean Vegetable Sandwich   SERVES 1

2 tablespoons yogurt spread	6 calamata olives, pitted
2 slices sprouted sesame bread	1 tablespoon fresh basil chiffonade
5 thin slices cucumber	1 piece fruit of your choice
3 slices tomato	

Spread the yogurt evenly onto each slice of bread. Layer with the cucumber, tomato, olives, and basil.

Serve with a piece of fruit for a light, refreshing lunch.

Pasta Primavera   SERVES 4

1 cup diced plum tomatoes	4 tablespoons medium-diced red onion
3 tablespoons fresh basil chiffonade	2 tablespoons julienned red bell pepper

1½ tablespoons minced garlic
4 tablespoons olive oil, plus more
    for the pasta
Salt and pepper
⅛ pound whole wheat pasta (any
    shape you prefer)

2 tablespoons julienned yellow bell
    pepper
2 tablespoons julienned zucchini
2 tablespoons julienned summer squash
Freshly grated Parmesan cheese, for
    serving

In a medium bowl, toss the tomatoes with 2 tablespoon of the basil, ¾ tablespoon of the garlic, 2 tablespoons of the olive oil, and salt and pepper to taste. Set aside.

Heat lightly salted water in a saucepan. Add the pasta and boil until al dente, about 10 minutes. Drain the pasta, but do not rinse. Toss the pasta lightly with tongs to allow the heat to escape; this prevents the pasta from sticking. Once the pasta is slightly cooled, drizzle a very small amount of oil over the pasta while still tossing to coat. Set aside the pasta.

Heat a large sauté pan over medium to high heat, then add the remaining 2 tablespoons of olive oil. Sauté the onion, then add the bell peppers and cook for about 1 minute, stirring constantly. Add the zucchini and squash and sauté for another minute, then add the remaining garlic and sauté quickly, being careful not to overcook. Next add the tomato mixture, then the pasta, being careful not to overcook the tomatoes. Heat everything through and add a little bit of water if needed to prevent sticking and drying. Remove from the heat after 2 minutes.

Season the dish with salt and pepper to taste and serve with the remaining tablespoon of fresh basil and some Parmesan.

Afternoon Snack

Select any of the snack options from the midmorning category or choose one from the following list.

Brown Rice Crackers and Carrots

5 brown rice crackers

5 carrot sticks

Celery Sticks with Tahini

3 3-inch-long celery sticks   1 tablespoon tahini

Use almond butter if you prefer.
   Dip the sticks and enjoy.

Dried Apricots

4 dried apricots

Banana with Berries

Half a banana   ½ cup blueberries

Fruit

1 medium apple, pear, or orange

Enjoy whole or sliced.
   Tip: Fruit is a great blood-sugar stabilizer in the later part of the day, when a quick pick-me-up is necessary.

Dinner

Grilled Turkey Burgers, Tarragon Mushroom Rice, and Corn   SERVES 1

6 ounces ground turkey   ⅓ cup sliced mushrooms
Drizzle of olive oil   ¼ cup jasmine rice
Salt and pepper   1 teaspoon dried tarragon
1 piece corn on the cob, husk on   ½ cup vegetable stock
½ tablespoon butter

Preheat the grill to 375°F.
   Form the turkey into a patty, drizzle it with olive oil, and season with a pinch of salt and pepper.

Soak the corncob, still in the husk, in cold water for 5 minutes, to prevent the husk from drying out completely while the corn steams.

In a small saucepan, melt the butter over medium heat. Add the mushrooms and sauté them for 3 to 5 minutes, until cooked. Add the rice and tarragon and sauté for 1 more minute. Pour in the vegetable stock, cover, and simmer for about 5 minutes.

Place the corn on the grill and rotate occasionally so the husk does not burn. Grill it until the husk is dry, 7 to 10 minutes.

Grill the turkey burger for 4 minutes on each side, making sure it is cooked through.

Remove the corn from the husk, place it on a plate with the rice and the turkey burger, and serve.

Soft Chicken Tacos SERVES 4

1 pound skinless, boneless chicken breasts
1 tablespoon olive oil
Salt and pepper
1 tablespoon coconut oil
Juice of ½ lime

8 medium whole wheat tortillas
Salsa fresca, for serving (optional)
Guacamole, for serving (optional)
Diced tomatoes, for serving (optional)
Shredded lettuce, for serving (optional)

Brush the chicken strips with the olive oil and then sprinkle with salt and pepper.

Place a skillet or a grill pan over high heat and coat with the coconut oil.

Cook the chicken 2 to 4 minutes per side, until cooked through. Set aside to cool for about 5 minutes.

Pour the lime juice over the cooked chicken.

Cut the chicken across the grain into 1-inch strips and then again into bite-size pieces.

Warm the tortillas by first sprinkling them with water, then placing them in a dry pan over low heat for about 2 minutes on each side. Use tongs to lift them out and wrap in a towel to keep warm.

Assemble the tacos with your desired add-ons—salsa, guacamole, diced tomatoes, and shredded lettuce—and serve.

Turkey Cutlets Parmesan   SERVES 4

1 ½ tablespoons olive oil
4 turkey cutlets (about 4 ounces each)
Salt and pepper
Flour, for dredging
1 clove garlic, thinly sliced

1 15-ounce can diced tomatoes,
   juice reserved
½ teaspoon dried oregano
¼ cup freshly grated Parmesan
   cheese

In a large nonstick skillet, heat 1 tablespoon of the olive oil over medium-high heat. While the oil is heating, season the turkey with salt and pepper and dredge in flour.

Sauté the turkey over medium-high heat until golden brown, about 2 minutes on each side. Transfer the turkey to a platter and cover to keep it warm.

Reduce the heat to medium, add the remaining ½ tablespoon oil and the garlic to the skillet, and cook until the garlic is lightly golden, about 1 minute. Add the tomatoes and their juice and the oregano and stir with a wooden spoon to release any caramelized bits that may be stuck to the pan. Season lightly with salt and pepper.

Add the turkey and any juices that have accumulated on the platter back to the pan. Simmer until the turkey is cooked through, about 10 minutes. Remove the turkey to a clean serving platter and cover to keep it warm.

Simmer the tomato mixture until it has reduced by half, about 5 minutes. Adjust the seasoning if needed.

Sprinkle the turkey with Parmesan cheese, spoon the tomatoes over the top, and serve.

Basic Beef Chili   SERVES 4

2 cloves garlic
2 teaspoons chili powder
1 teaspoon pepper
1 teaspoon salt
1 ½ cups chopped tomatoes
1 tablespoon olive oil

1 pound ground beef sirloin
1 onion, chopped
3 cups low-sodium beef broth
1 16-ounce can kidney beans,
   drained and rinsed

Combine the garlic, chili powder, pepper, salt, and ½ cup of the tomatoes in a food processor and pulse to blend. Set aside.

In a large skillet or soup pot, heat the olive oil over high heat. Add the ground sirloin and brown it, breaking the meat into small chunks with a wooden spoon as it cooks. Add the onion, reduce the heat to medium, and cook for 5 minutes. Add the tomato mixture and cook for 5 more minutes. Add the remaining tomatoes and the broth and simmer for 30 minutes. Add the kidney beans, heat thoroughly, and serve.

Basic Turkey Chili   SERVES 4

2 cloves garlic
2 tablespoons chili powder
1 teaspoon pepper
1 teaspoon salt
1½ cups chopped tomatoes
1 tablespoon olive oil

1 pound ground lean turkey
1 onion, chopped
3 cups low-sodium chicken broth
1 16-ounce can kidney beans,
    drained and rinsed

Combine the garlic, chili powder, pepper, salt, and ½ cup of the tomatoes in a food processor and pulse to blend. Set aside.

In a large skillet or soup pot, heat the olive oil over high heat. Add the ground turkey and brown it, breaking the meat into small chunks with a wooden spoon as it cooks. Add the onion, reduce the heat to medium, and cook for 5 minutes. Add the tomato mixture and cook for 5 more minutes. Add the remaining tomatoes and the broth and simmer for 30 minutes. Add the kidney beans, heat thoroughly, and serve.

Chicken and Asparagus with Dijon Sauce   SERVES 4

1 tablespoon olive oil
1 pound skinless, boneless chicken
    breasts
Salt and pepper
1 pound asparagus, cut into
    2-inch pieces
1 small onion, minced

Olive oil spray
1 clove garlic, minced
½ cup dry white wine
1 cup low-sodium chicken broth
2 tablespoons Dijon mustard
½ cup fat-free sour cream
2 tablespoons chopped tarragon

In a large sauté pan, heat the olive oil over medium-high heat.
Season the chicken breasts with salt and pepper and add them to

the pan in a single layer. Sauté the chicken on both sides until golden brown, about 2 minutes per side. Transfer the chicken to a platter and cover to keep it warm.

Place the asparagus in a microwave-safe bowl with a splash of water and cover it loosely with plastic wrap. Microwave the asparagus on high until it is just tender, 2 to 3 minutes. Drain and set aside.

Place the onion in a sauté pan and spritz with olive oil spray and cook over medium-high heat until it is soft and translucent, about 5 minutes. Add the garlic and cook for 1 minute more. Add the wine to the pan, lower the heat to medium, and cook until the wine is reduced by half (about 15 minutes). Add the chicken broth and again reduce the mixture by half. Whisk in the mustard, sour cream, and 1 tablespoon of the tarragon and stir until the sauce is smooth and creamy. Add the chicken and asparagus to the sauce to heat for a minute or two.

Transfer the chicken and asparagus to a platter, sprinkle with the remaining tablespoon of tarragon, and serve.

Chicken Burritos   SERVES 4

For the salsa
⅔ small onion onion, chopped
1 10-ounce can diced tomatoes, drained
1½ cloves garlic
¾ jalapeño pepper, seeded
2½ tablespoons chopped fresh cilantro leaves
⅔ cup water
Pinch of sugar
Salt and pepper

For the burritos
4 large whole wheat tortillas
⅔ pound skinless, boneless chicken breasts
2 teaspoons olive oil
Salt and pepper
½ cup fat-free sour cream, for serving (optional)
⅔ cup water
¼ cup fresh cilantro leaves, chopped, for serving (optional)

To make the salsa: Combine all the salsa ingredients in a small saucepan and bring to a boil, then reduce the heat to a simmer and cook until half of the liquid evaporates, about 15 minutes. Turn off the heat and let cool uncovered for another 15 minutes. Pour the mixture into a blender and puree. Cover and chill in the refrigerator for about 15 minutes.

To make the burritos: Preheat the oven to 350°F.

Wrap the tortillas in foil and warm them in the oven for about 10 minutes.

Preheat a skillet or a grill pan to medium high.

Brush the chicken breasts with the olive oil, then season with salt and pepper. Cook the chicken until the juices run clear and the chicken is cooked through, about 6 minutes per side. Transfer the chicken to a cutting board and let rest for a few minutes before slicing it into thin strips or chopping it into small pieces.

Fill the tortillas with chicken slices, salsa, and your preferred garnishes and serve.

Grilled Chicken Spinach Salad with Raspberry-Balsamic Vinaigrette SERVES 4

For the dressing
2 tablespoons olive oil
½ cup red raspberry jam
1 tablespoon Dijon mustard
1½ tablespoons balsamic vinegar

For the salad
4 pregrilled skinless, boneless chicken breasts (4 to 6 ounces each), sliced into ½-inch-thick strips
8 cups baby spinach leaves
1 red bell pepper, julienned
1 cup diced mushrooms
½ cup thinly sliced red onion
2 hard-boiled eggs (yolk removed and discarded), chopped

To make the dressing: In a small saucepan, heat the olive oil over medium heat. Add the jam, mustard, and balsamic vinegar and heat thoroughly (do not boil).

To prepare the salad: In a large bowl, toss the chicken, spinach, and bell pepper with the warm dressing.

Divide the chicken mixture among four large serving plates, sprinkle with the mushrooms, onions, and egg whites, and serve.

Chicken and Artichokes   SERVES 4

1 tablespoon olive oil
1 small onion, chopped
2 cloves garlic, minced
1 9-ounce bag frozen artichoke
   hearts, thawed and quartered
1 cup sliced mushrooms
1 red bell pepper, seeded and
   sliced into 1/4-inch strips

Salt and pepper
4 skinless, boneless chicken breasts
   (4 to 6 ounces each), sliced
   into 1/2-inch-thick strips
1 teaspoon chopped fresh rosemary
1/4 cup dry white wine
1 cup low-sodium chicken broth

Preheat the oven to 350°F.

In a large skillet, heat the olive oil over medium heat. Add the onion and cook, stirring occasionally, until it is soft and translucent, about 5 minutes. Add the garlic, artichoke hearts, mushrooms, and bell pepper, season with salt and pepper, and cook for 2 more minutes. Set aside.

Season the chicken pieces with the rosemary and salt and pepper and place them in a large baking dish in a single layer. Spoon the artichoke mixture evenly over the chicken and add the wine and broth. Cook the chicken until the internal temperature is 165°F, as indicated by a meat thermometer inserted into the thickest part of the chicken (18 to 20 minutes). Remove the chicken from the oven and allow to cool for 5 minutes before serving.

Beef and Mushroom Stroganoff   SERVES 4

1 pound lean beef sirloin, sliced thin
Salt and pepper
1 1/2 tablespoons olive oil
1/2 large or 1 small onion, sliced
1 pound fresh mushrooms, sliced
1 clove garlic, minced

1 cup nonfat sour cream
1/2 cup chopped tomatoes
   (canned or fresh)
1/2 teaspoon hot sauce
2 cups cooked, hot egg noodles

Season the sirloin with salt and pepper. In a large skillet, heat the olive oil over high heat. Add the sirloin and brown on both sides, about 8 minutes total. Set the sirloin on a plate and cover to keep it warm.

Reduce the heat to medium and add the onion. Season lightly with salt and pepper and cook, stirring occasionally, until the onion begins to soften, about 5 minutes. Add the mushrooms and cook until soft, about 7 minutes. Add the garlic and cook for 1 minute. Reduce the heat to low and add the sour cream, tomatoes, and hot sauce, combining well and heating thoroughly. Return the sirloin to the pan along with any juices. Adjust the seasonings if needed.

Divide the egg noodles among four plates, arranging them in a small ring on the plate, leaving a hole in the center. Spoon some of the beef mixture into the center of each ring and serve.

Meat Loaf with Garlic Smashed Potatoes   SERVES 4

For the meat loaf
1 tablespoon olive oil
1 medium onion, chopped
2 cloves garlic, minced
5 tablespoons ketchup, plus more
   for brushing on the loaf
1 large egg
1 cup bread crumbs
2 tablespoons chopped fresh parsley
1/4 teaspoon salt
1/4 teaspoon freshly ground black pepper
1/2 pound lean ground turkey
1/2 pound lean ground beef sirloin

For the potatoes
1 whole garlic bulb, unpeeled
Olive oil
1 pound Yukon Gold potatoes
1 cup low-sodium chicken broth
Salt and pepper

To make the meat loaf: Preheat the oven to 350°F.

In a skillet, heat the olive oil over medium heat. Add the onion and cook for 5 minutes. Add the garlic and cook for 2 minutes more. Set aside and cool.

In a large bowl, thoroughly combine the ketchup, egg, bread crumbs, parsley, salt, pepper, and the cooled onion mixture. Add the turkey and beef sirloin and mix until just combined. Pack the mixture into a greased 9-inch loaf pan, brush the top with ketchup, and bake for approximately 1 hour, until fully cooked. Once the center is cooked through (you can test for doneness with a fork or by using a meat thermometer inserted into the thickest part of the meat—it should read 170°F), remove the meat loaf from the oven and let stand for 10 minutes before slicing.

To make the potatoes: Preheat the oven to 350°F.

Place the garlic bulb in an ovenproof dish and drizzle with olive oil. Place the dish, uncovered, in the oven for 15 to 20 minutes, until the garlic is golden brown and soft. Remove from the oven and let it cool.

Prick each potato several times with the tip of a sharp knife. Place them in a single layer in a microwave-safe container and microwave until tender, about 8 to 10 minutes depending on the size of the potatoes.

In a small saucepan, bring the stock to a boil, then reduce the heat to a simmer.

Meanwhile, squeeze the cooled roasted garlic bulb over a small bowl to release each clove of garlic. Mash the garlic with a fork and throw away the skins.

Mash the potatoes (and their skins) with a potato masher or a fork. Add the roasted garlic and mix thoroughly. Slowly add the stock until the desired consistency is reached. Season with salt and pepper to taste.

Serve the potatoes with a slice of the meat loaf.

Beef Tenderloin with Roasted Vegetables

SERVES 4

4 small red potatoes, halved
2 carrots, peeled and cut into
  ¾-inch pieces
2 parsnips, peeled and cut into
  ¾-inch pieces

2 tablespoons olive oil
1 tablespoon chopped fresh rosemary,
  or 1 teaspoon dried
Salt and pepper
1 pound beef tenderloin

Preheat the oven to 425°F.

In a medium bowl, toss the potatoes, carrots, and parsnips with the olive oil, rosemary, salt, and pepper. Transfer the vegetables to a shallow roasting pan and bake for 10 minutes.

Season the beef with salt and a generous amount of pepper. Remove the vegetables from the oven and place the beef on top of them in the roasting pan. Return the pan to the oven and cook

the vegetables and beef for 15 minutes. Reduce the oven temperature to 350°F and continue roasting for an additional 15 minutes,
or until the vegetables are tender and the beef is cooked to the
desired doneness (to check for doneness, insert a meat thermometer into the thickest part of the roast; it should read 135°F for
medium rare).

Let the tenderloin rest for 10 minutes before slicing.

Serve a few slices of the beef with a large spoonful of the vegetables.

Marinated Grilled Flank Steak with Cherry Tomatoes and Basil   SERVES 4

2 cloves garlic, minced	Salt and pepper
3 shallots, minced	1½ pounds flank steak
1 tablespoon light brown sugar	1 pint cherry tomatoes, halved
1 tablespoon Worcestershire sauce	¼ cup finely sliced red onion
⅓ cup dry red wine	1 tablespoon chopped fresh basil
¼ cup balsamic vinegar	1 tablespoon red wine vinegar
Olive oil	1 tablespoon extra-virgin olive oil

In a medium bowl, combine the garlic, shallots, sugar, Worcestershire
sauce, wine, balsamic vinegar, and olive oil. Add salt and pepper to
taste.

Place the flank steak in a shallow bowl and pour the marinade
over it, then cover and refrigerate for 1 hour or overnight.

Preheat the grill to high.

Remove the flank steak from the marinade and discard the marinade.

Grill the flank steak for 4 to 8 minutes on each side, depending on
the desired doneness. Let the steak rest on a carving board for 4 to 5
minutes before slicing.

Meanwhile, combine the cherry tomatoes, onion, basil, red wine
vinegar, and extra-virgin olive oil in a small bowl. Season with salt
and pepper and set aside (the tomatoes can be prepared ahead of
time and stored in the refrigerator).

Slice the steak on the bias and serve with the cherry tomatoes.

Mixed-Up Beef with Sugar Snap Peas and Crybaby Carrots   SERVES 4

1 tablespoon light soy sauce
2 teaspoons grated fresh ginger
3 cloves garlic, minced
1/2 teaspoon red chili paste
3 tablespoons dry sherry or water
1 pound flank steak, sliced across the
  grain into 2-inch pieces

18 baby carrots, quartered
1/2 pound sugar snap or snow peas
2 teaspoons peanut oil
1/2 cup low-sodium beef broth
1 tablespoon cornstarch

In a small bowl, combine the soy sauce, ginger, garlic, chili paste, and sherry. Set the flank steak in a shallow bowl and pour the marinade over the meat. Cover and refrigerate the steak for at least 10 minutes or up to 1 hour.

Bring a medium pot of water to a boil. Toss in the carrots and parboil for about 2 minutes, then quickly remove them with a slotted spoon. Set aside.

Add the peas to the water and parboil for 1 minute. Set the peas aside. Drain the pot, refill with cold water, and set aside.

Remove the beef from the marinade, let the excess drip off, and discard the marinade.

Heat a wok or a frying pan over high heat and add the peanut oil. Stir-fry the beef until just cooked on all sides, about 2 minutes. Add the carrots and peas to the pan and toss. Add the beef broth and simmer for 3 minutes. Mix the cornstarch with 2 tablespoons of water until smooth, add it to the beef mixture, and simmer for 3 minutes.

Cook until the sauce thickens, about 2 minutes.

Serve in a bowl and enjoy.

Pan-Seared Sirloin Steaks with Yukon Gold Potatoes   SERVES 4

8 small Yukon Gold potatoes or
  red-skinned potatoes, halved
6 teaspoons olive oil
Salt and pepper

1 small yellow onion, chopped
1/4 cup red wine or balsamic vinegar
1 15-ounce can diced tomatoes, juice
  reserved

| 4 top sirloin steaks (about 4 ounces each) | 8 black olives, pitted and halved |
| | Freshly shaved Parmesan cheese, for serving |

Place the potatoes in a microwave-safe dish and microwave until tender, about 5 minutes.

In a nonstick skillet, heat 1 teaspoon of the olive oil over high heat.

Add the potatoes, cut side down, and season liberally with salt and pepper.

When the potatoes are well browned (about 20 minutes), remove to a dish and cover to keep warm.

Meanwhile, in a skillet large enough to accommodate all the steaks in a single layer, heat 3 teaspoons of the olive oil over high heat.

Season the steaks with salt and pepper and sear them in the hot skillet on both sides to the desired doneness, 2 to 3 minutes per side for medium rare.

Transfer the steaks to a plate and cover to keep warm.

Reduce the heat to medium and add the remaining 2 teaspoons of olive oil and the onion.

Cook the onion until it softens and begins to color, 3 to 4 minutes.

Add the wine and cook until the liquid has almost completely evaporated. Add the olives and tomatoes with their juices and simmer for 2 minutes.

Serve the steaks topped with a few shavings of the Parmesan and a large dollop of the tomato relish and the potatoes on the side.

Grilled Rosemary Tuna Steak over Garden Vegetable Salad   SERVES 1

6 ounces tuna steak	1/4 cup chopped jicama
1 tablespoon olive oil	1/8 cup chopped celery
1 teaspoon chopped garlic	1/8 cup shredded carrot
1 teaspoon chopped fresh rosemary	1/8 cup chopped green onion, white and green parts
Salt and pepper	3 cups mixed greens
1/4 cup chopped red bell pepper	1/2 lemon
1/4 cup chopped cucumber	

Put the tuna steak in a bowl with ½ tablespoon of the olive oil, the garlic, rosemary, and a pinch of salt and pepper. Cover and refrigerate for 1 hour. Discard the marinade.

Preheat the grill to 400°F. Grill the tuna steak for 2 minutes on each side. If you prefer it to be done a little more, cook it for 3 minutes on each side. Be careful: tuna steak cooks and dries out quickly.

Place all the other remaining ingredients except the lemon in a bowl. Squeeze the lemon over the vegetables, season with a pinch of salt and pepper, and toss.

Set the salad on a plate, top it with the sliced tuna steak, and enjoy.

Broiled Sole with Brussels Sprouts and Fingerling Potatoes SERVES 1

1 6-ounce sole filet
½ tablespoon butter
Salt and pepper
½ lemon

½ cup Brussels sprouts, halved
5 fingerling potatoes, halved
½ tablespoon dried tarragon
1 tablespoon olive oil

Place the sole in an oven-safe pan. Melt the butter and drizzle it over the sole. Squeeze the lemon over the sole and season lightly with salt and pepper. Set aside.

Preheat the oven to 350°F.

Steam the Brussels sprouts in a medium pot with about 2 inches of water so that the Brussels sprouts just barely float. Steam on high heat for 8 minutes, or until the sprouts are bright green and slightly soft. Remove them from the pot, drain the water, and set aside.

In another medium pot, boil the potatoes for 15 minutes, or until they are slightly soft when poked with a fork. Remove the potatoes from the pot, drain the water, and set aside to cool. In a medium bowl, toss the potatoes with the tarragon, a pinch of salt and pepper, and ½ tablespoon of the olive oil until the potatoes are coated evenly.

Spread out the potatoes in one layer in a roasting pan. Bake them for 15 minutes, or until golden brown. Remove the potatoes from the oven and cover to keep them warm.

Set the oven to broil and place the fish in a shallow ceramic or glass casserole dish and broil for 3 to 4 minutes. Sole cooks very quickly, so watch it carefully.

In a small sauté pan, heat the remaining ½ tablespoon of olive oil over medium heat and sauté the Brussels sprouts with a pinch of salt and pepper for 3 minutes until light brown.

Place the fish, potatoes, and Brussels sprouts on a large plate and enjoy.

Mediterranean Chicken Pasta with Sambuca Reduction SERVES 2

2 tablespoons olive oil, plus more
   for the chicken
8 ounces skinless, boneless chicken
   breast, sliced into ¼-inch strips
Salt and pepper
2 (medium cap) portabella
   mushrooms, sliced
1 tablespoon minced fresh garlic

4 tablespoons Sambuca
½ cup chicken or vegetable stock
¼ pound cooked linguini, cooled
½ pound arugula
6 ounces fresh mozzarella, chopped
   into ½-inch cubes
2 teaspoon oregano

Drizzle olive oil lightly over the chicken to coat and sprinkle it with salt and pepper.

Heat a sauté pan, then add the 2 tablespoons of olive oil and the chicken. Cook the chicken on medium-high heat, tilting the pan to ensure that the entire surface is coated with oil. Turn the chicken over after 8 minutes; add the mushrooms and sauté for 2 to 4 minutes, until the mushrooms are cooked through. Add the garlic and sauté for 1 minute. Pull the pan away from the stove and add the Sambuca to deglaze the pan. Return the pan to the heat. Cook the alcohol off for 1 minute, then add the stock and simmer for 15 minutes.

Toss in the pasta, and reduce the sauce into the pasta for 2 minutes. Add the arugula and toss lightly, then turn off the heat and toss in the fresh mozzarella and oregano.

Using tongs, remove the linguini to a bowl and twirl the pasta into a mound. Top with the chicken, vegetables, and sauce and serve.

Brown Rice Pasta with Shiitake Mushrooms, Caramelized Onions, and Spinach   SERVES 1

1 teaspoon butter
½ cup onion, sliced ¼ inch thick
½ cup brown rice pasta (any shape you prefer)
1 tablespoon olive oil
2 tablespoons diced shallots
1 cup shiitake mushrooms, sliced ½ inch thick

2 tablespoons chopped fresh rosemary
3 cups baby spinach
1 cup vegetable stock
Salt and pepper
1 tablespoon freshly grated Parmesan

Heat the butter in a small sauté pan over medium heat. Add the onions and sauté until they begin to turn translucent, 2 to 3 minutes. Reduce the heat to low and continue to cook the onions, stirring occasionally, until they caramelize (they will have a light brown caramel color), about 3 minutes. Set the onions aside.

Bring salted water to a boil and cook the pasta according to the package instructions. Make sure the pasta is a bit al dente. Set the pasta aside.

In a large sauté pan, heat the olive oil over medium heat. Add the shallots and sauté for 1 minute.

Add the mushrooms and 1 tablespoon of the rosemary and sauté, stirring constantly, for 3 minutes. Once the mushrooms are wilted, add the onions and spinach; sauté for 1 more minute, until the spinach wilts. Add the vegetable stock and a pinch of salt and pepper and simmer for about 5 minutes.

Then add the pasta and simmer until the sauce is absorbed into the pasta, making sure not to dry out the sauce but rather reduce it to a thin consistency, about 5 minutes. The sauce should be light, not soupy.

Add the remaining tablespoon of rosemary and taste the sauce to see if you need more salt and pepper—this dish is great with a little extra pepper.

Place the pasta in a bowl and neatly arrange the vegetables on top. Garnish with the Parmesan cheese and enjoy.

Tip: Brown rice pasta is a great alternative to wheat-based pasta and is packed with great protein.

Oven Roasted Vegetables with Tomato-Chickpea Rice

SERVES 1

1 small zucchini, sliced ½ inch
   thick
2 ½ × 3-inch slices summer squash
3 3 × 1-inch slices red bell pepper
2 large broccoli florets
1 tablespoon olive oil

Salt and pepper
1 tablespoon chopped onion
¼ cup diced tomato
¼ cup basmati rice
1 tablespoon herbes de Provence
¼ cup chickpeas

In a medium bowl, toss the zucchini, squash, bell pepper, and broccoli with ½ tablespoon of the olive oil and season with salt and pepper until the vegetables are evenly coated.

Preheat the oven to 400°F.

In a small saucepan, heat the remaining ½ tablespoon of olive oil over medium heat. Sauté the onions until transparent (about 2 minutes), then add the tomatoes. Cook for 2 minutes, then add the rice, stir, and cook for 1 minute. Add ½ cup of water, the herbes de Provence, and a pinch of salt and pepper.

Cover the rice and reduce the heat to low. Place the vegetables on a baking sheet and roast in the oven for 20 minutes, rotating the tray once to ensure even cooking.

When the rice is halfway cooked, about 4 minutes, stir in the chickpeas and cover again for 4 minutes.

Place the rice on the center of a plate and the vegetables around the rice and enjoy.

Lemon-Dill Halibut with Asparagus and Mixed Greens

SERVES 1

6 ounces halibut
1 tablespoon olive oil
1 teaspoon fresh dill
Salt and pepper

6 spears asparagus
1 cup mixed salad greens
½ fresh lemon

Place the halibut in an oven-safe pan, drizzle with ½ tablespoon of the olive oil, sprinkle with dill, lightly season with salt and pepper. Cut the lemon in half and squeeze one of the quarters over the halibut. Reserve the other quarter of lemon.

Preheat the broiler. Place the asparagus in another oven-safe pan, drizzle with the remaining ½ tablespoon of olive oil, and lightly sprinkle with salt and pepper.

Broil both the halibut and the asparagus for 5 minutes, rotating the asparagus once to ensure even cooking.

Place the salad greens on a plate, top with the fish and the asparagus—which will wilt the greens slightly—then squeeze the remaining lemon quarter over the plate and enjoy.

Grilled Beef Tenderloin, Broccoli, and Brown Rice   SERVES 1

6 ounces beef tenderloin
1 tablespoon olive oil
Seasoning salt
½ cup brown rice

1 cup vegetable broth
½ cup broccoli florets
1 teaspoon butter
Salt and pepper

Place the tenderloin in a bowl with the olive oil and sprinkle with seasoning salt, making sure to lightly coat the entire piece of beef.

In a small saucepan, cook the brown rice with the vegetable broth over low heat, covered, for 30 minutes.

Preheat the grill to 375°F. Place the tenderloin on the grill. For medium rare, cook for 4 minutes on each side. Check the internal temperature with a meat thermometer inserted into the thickest part of the meat—145°F for medium rare.

In a steamer (follow the manufacturer's instructions) or in a small pan with just enough water to cover the broccoli, steam the broccoli, then drain (not necessary if you used a steamer) and lightly toss with the butter and salt and pepper.

Place the rice, tenderloin, and broccoli on a plate and enjoy.

Grilled Sesame Salmon with Braised Baby Bok Choy

SERVES 1

1 6-ounce wild salmon filet
2 tablespoons sesame
   seeds
1 tablespoon sesame oil

2 stalks baby bok choy, sliced in
   half and washed thoroughly
1 teaspoon fresh basil chiffonade
Salt (optional)

Place the salmon in a bowl with the sesame seeds and ½ tablespoon of the sesame oil and toss lightly to coat the salmon evenly.

Preheat the grill to 375°F. Place the salmon on the grill and cook for 4 minutes on each side. (If you prefer salmon rare, reduce the cooking time to 3 minutes on each side.)

In a medium sauté pan over medium heat, steam the baby bok choy with 2 ounces of water, covered, for 2 minutes. Drain the water; add the remaining ½ tablespoon of sesame oil and the basil and sauté for 1 minute. If desired, add a pinch of salt.

Place the salmon and the bok choy on a plate and enjoy.

Roasted Chicken and Vegetables   SERVES 1

½ chicken, bone-in
1½ tablespoons olive oil
1 tablespoon fresh chopped oregano
1 tablespoon fresh chopped rosemary
1 tablespoon fresh chopped sage
1 teaspoon minced garlic

Salt and pepper
½ red bell pepper, cut lengthwise
   into 4¾-inch-thick pieces
½ cup summer squash, sliced
   ½ inch thick

Preheat the oven to 350°F.

Place the chicken in a roasting pan and rub with 1 tablespoon of the olive oil, the herbs, the garlic, and salt and pepper.

Toss the bell peppers and summer squash in a bowl with the remaining ½ tablespoon of olive oil and a pinch of salt and pepper, then place the vegetables on a separate roasting pan or baking sheet.

Roast the chicken for 30 minutes, or until the internal temperature is 165°F, as indicated by a meat thermometer inserted into the thickest part of the chicken.

Remove the chicken from the oven, raise the heat to 375°F, and roast the vegetables for 10 minutes.

While the vegetables are roasting, allow the chicken to rest for 5 minutes and then slice the meat off the bones.

Remove the vegetables from the oven, plate them with the chicken, and enjoy.

Spinach Sauté with Garlic and Parmesan Cheese SERVES 4

1 teaspoon olive oil
1 teaspoon crushed garlic
4 cups spinach leaves, washed

Salt and pepper
1 tablespoon freshly grated
Parmesan cheese

In a large skillet, heat the olive oil over medium-low heat.

Add the garlic and cook for 1 minute. Add the spinach and salt and pepper and toss with the olive oil and the garlic until the spinach just begins to wilt, about 1 minute.

Remove from the skillet, sprinkle with Parmesan cheese, and serve.

8

Star Quality Exercises

Environment/Terrain-Based and Weather-Based Cardio Choices

For your basic cardio workout, use the great outdoors as your gym and you are less likely to grow bored and give up. Here's what you can do outside.

In the mountains: Hike, jog, power walk, rock climb, bike, ski, snowboard, snowshoe, ice skate, cross-country ski, mountain climb

At the beach: Swim, jog in place in the water, run on the shore in shin-to-knee-deep water, walk or jog in soft sand, alternate swimming and running in the water, kayak, do aqua aerobics, kick with a flutter board, surf, paddle board, wake board, waterski, windsurf, canoe, in-line skate

In the city: Jog, power walk, run, climb stairs, bike, in-line skate

In the country: Jog, power walk, run, bike

Add Some Glitter to Your Cardio and Resistance Exercises

Each day you work out, you will do a minimum of twenty minutes of aerobic exercise. Because variation helps to maintain interest, following is an array of options for accessorizing your basic cardio workout that you can do anywhere. Take it outside for an exciting, ever-changing, Star Quality fitness routine.

You can accessorize your resistance routine to help create a constantly evolving and personalized fitness program that will help you shape your ideal movie-star physique. Change it often to shake things up, engage different muscles, shape your body faster, and stay interested. At the beginning of each week I will let you know how many upper-body and lower-body resistance moves you should do. Use the resistance exercises described in this chapter to make your selection.

You will notice that there are designated reps and weights for each body type: Naomi-type (a dancer's body), Demi-type (a movie star's body), and Madonna-type (an athlete's body). This is because each body type requires a slightly different fitness regimen in order to target problem areas, utilize built-in strength, and maximize its potential.

Essential Extras

You will need the following:

Good cardio sneakers

Running shoes

Cardio shoes are meant to give you stability. They do not propel your body forward in a running or walking motion. They have more support on the sides of your feet to help you maintain your balance. Wear your cardio shoes when doing your resistance training.

Running shoes help propel your body forward. They have very little support on the sides of your feet.

If you plan to go out and run and then do your resistance training at your destination, select hybrid exercise shoes, also known as cross-trainers (ask a salesperson what shoe is most appropriate for your feet and activities).

Wearing the right shoes can help minimize injuries and maximize your workout.

You may need any or all of these items:

Masking tape

A chair or a bench

A yoga or other mat

A yardstick

A pen or a pencil

Paper

A heart-rate monitor (unless you know how to accurately check your pulse)

A stool or a step

A fitness ball

2-pound (beginner), 5-pound (beginner), 10-pound (intermediate), and 15-pound (advanced) hand weights (the size you'll use will be based on the exercise and your fitness level)

What's with the free weights and fitness ball if this is an outdoor workout? Some basic accessories can make specific exercises more effective. If I could translate an exercise to be exclusively outdoor—equipment free—I did, but with some arm and leg exercises, you will appreciate the extra challenge provided by some basic equipment.

Single-Arm Bent-Over Row

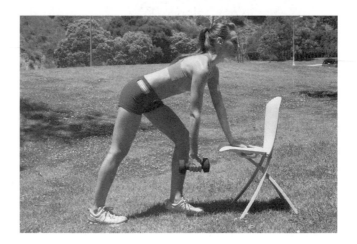

Naomi-type	8–12 reps
Demi-type	10–15 reps
Madonna-type	15–20 reps
Beginner	5-lb weight
Intermediate	10-lb weight
Advanced	15-lb weight

POSITION
- Stand in front of a chair or a bench.
- Bend forward at your torso and allow your left hand to rest on the chair.
- Keep your right leg straight at the knee, but allow a slight bend in the hip.
- Keep your back straight and long.
- Balance your body weight between your left knee and your right leg.
- Your arms should be straight.
- Hold a dumbbell in your right hand with your palm facing your legs.

MOVEMENT
- Keeping your right arm close to your body, bend your elbow, lifting the weight and bringing your elbow up to touch your torso.
- Keep your forearm perpendicular to the ground. Your forearm should move up and down only while your upper arm moves back to meet the angle of your back.
- Your arm should bend to a 90-degree angle as you move your elbow.
- Slowly and with control, lower your arm to a straight position.
- Repeat until you complete one set, then repeat on the other side.

Seated Bent-Over
Row, Elbows In

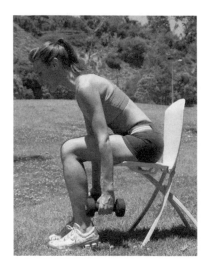

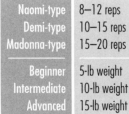

Naomi-type	8–12 reps
Demi-type	10–15 reps
Madonna-type	15–20 reps
Beginner	5-lb weight
Intermediate	10-lb weight
Advanced	15-lb weight

POSITION

- Sit on a bench or a chair and place a dumbell next to each of your feet.
- Bend forward at your waist so that your torso rests on your quads.
- Keep your back straight and your neck in line with your back.
- Let your arms drop down straight to the ground.
- Hold the dumbbells with your palms facing your legs.

MOVEMENT

- Keeping your arms close to your body and without letting your back or your neck curve, bend your elbows, lifting the dumbbells and bringing your elbows up to touch your torso.
- Keep your forearms perpendicular to the ground. Your forearms should only move up and down while your upper arms move back to meet the angle of your back.
- Your arm should bend to a 90-degree angle as you move your elbows.
- Slowly and with control, lower your arms to a straight position.
- Repeat until you complete one set.

Seated Bent-Over Row, Elbows Out

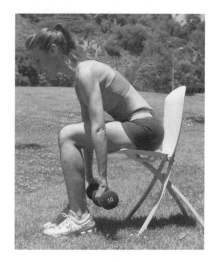

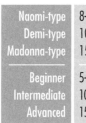

Naomi-type	8–12 reps
Demi-type	10–15 reps
Madonna-type	15–20 reps
Beginner	5-lb weight
Intermediate	10-lb weight
Advanced	15-lb weight

POSITION
- Sit on a bench or a chair and place a dumbell next to each of your feet.
- Bend forward at your waist so that your torso rests on your quads.
- Keep your back straight and your neck in line with your back.
- Let your arms drop down straight to the ground.
- Hold the dumbbells with your palms facing your legs.

MOVEMENT
- Keeping your arms away from your body and without letting your back or neck curve, bend your elbows, lifting the dumbbells and bringing your elbows up and out.
- Keep your forearms perpendicular to the ground. Your forearms should only move up and down while your upper arms move back to meet the angle of your back.
- Your arms should bend to a 90-degree angle as you move your elbows.
- Slowly and with control, lower your arms to a straight position.
- Repeat until you complete one set.

Lying-Down Pull-Up, Overhand Grip

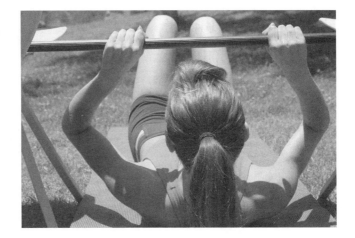

Naomi-type	8–12 reps
Demi-type	10–15 reps
Madonna-type	15–20 reps

POSITION
- You will need two sturdy chairs set approximately 3 feet apart.
- Place a broomstick or another sturdy stick that can hold your weight across the chairs.
- Lie on your back on a mat between the chairs so that the stick is above your chest.
- Your knees should be bent, with your feet flat on the ground.
- Grab the stick with an overhand grip so that the tops of your hands are facing your head and your palms are facing your feet.
- Your hands should be shoulder-width apart.

MOVEMENT
- Engage your back, biceps, and triceps and pull your chest up toward the stick, lifting your back off the ground.
- Keep your back straight and lift your chest until it is approximately 3 inches from the stick.
- Slowly and with control, lower your body back down to the ground.
- Repeat until you complete one set.

Lying-Down Pull-Up, Underhand Grip

Naomi-type	8–12 reps
Demi-type	10–15 reps
Madonna-type	15–20 reps

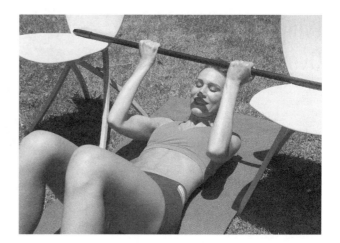

POSITION
- You will need two sturdy chairs set approximately 3 feet apart.
- Place a broomstick or another sturdy stick that can hold your weight across the chairs.
- Lie on your back on a mat between the chairs so that the stick is above your chest.
- Your knees should be bent, with your feet flat on the ground.
- Grab the stick with an underhand grip so that the backs of your hands are facing your feet and your palms are facing your head.
- Your hands should be shoulder-width apart.

MOVEMENT
- Engage your back, biceps, and triceps and pull your chest up toward the stick, lifting your back off the ground.
- Keep your back straight and lift your chest until it is approximately 3 inches from the stick.
- Slowly and with control, lower your body back down to the ground.
- Repeat until you complete one set.

Standard Push-Up

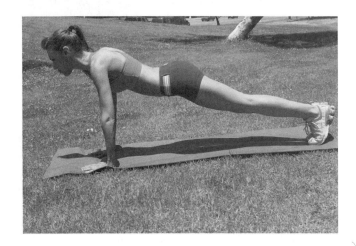

Naomi-type	8–12 reps
Demi-type	10–15 reps
Madonna-type	25–30 reps

POSITION
- Lie flat on your stomach on a mat.
- Place your hands flat on the ground 2 inches wider than your shoulders at your chest level.
- Your elbows should be bent at a 90-degree angle.
- Your knees should be straight with your feet flexed so that your toes are pushing down into the ground and your shins and knees are elevated.

MOVEMENT
- Engage your glutes, quads, abs, and arms and, with a straight body, raise yourself, straightening your elbows.
- Keep your body straight, from the top of your head to your toes. Do not let your butt sink or your knees bend.
- Once your arms are straight and you reach the top position, slowly and with control, lower your body by bending your elbows until they are at a 90-degree angle.
- *Do not* lower down completely onto the ground. Keep your body a few inches above the ground, then repeat, pushing your elbows straight and rising back up.
- Repeat until you complete one set.

Bent-Knee Push-Up

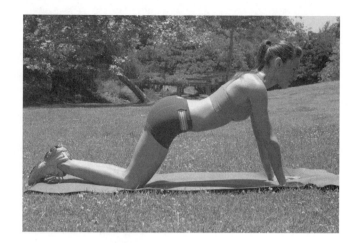

Naomi-type	8–12 reps
Demi-type	10–15 reps
Madonna-type	25–30 reps

POSITION

- Start on all fours on a mat with your back flat and parallel to the ground, your arms slightly bent to avoid locking your elbows, and your hands placed flat on the ground 2 inches wider than your shoulders.
- Bend your knees 90 degrees so that the bottoms of your feet are facing up.
- Maintain a straight line through your glutes and down the back of your hamstrings to your knees. You are now supporting your body with your hands and knees.

MOVEMENT

- Engage your glutes, quads, abs, and arms and, with a straight upper body, slowly and with control, bend your elbows to lower your body until your elbows are bent at a 90-degree angle.
- Keep your body straight, from the top of your head to your knees. Do not let your butt sink or your back arch.
- Once your arms are bent 90 degrees and you reach the bottom position, slowly and with control, straighten your arms and raise your body back to the starting position.
- Repeat until you complete one set.

Bench Press

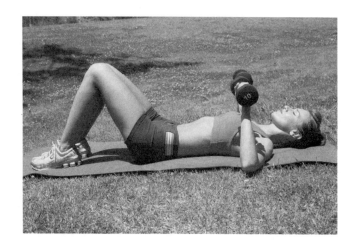

Naomi-type	8–12 reps
Demi-type	10–15 reps
Madonna-type	15–20 reps
Beginner	5-lb weight
Intermediate	10-lb weight
Advanced	15-lb weight

POSITION

- Lie on your back on a mat.
- Bend your knees and place your feet flat on the ground.
- Bend your elbows 90 degrees, folding your forearms back so that the tops of your hands fall on your shoulders.
- Your elbows should be at shoulder level with your elbows and triceps resting on the ground.
- Hold the dumbbells with your palms facing your hips.

MOVEMENT

- Engage your chest, arms, and back and press the dumbbells straight up above your chest.
- Press until your arms are straight, without locking your elbows.
- One you reach the top position, slowly and with control, lower your hands to the starting position.
- Be sure you lower your arms all the way down until your elbows and triceps are again resting on the ground.
- Repeat until you complete one set.

Dumbbell Fly

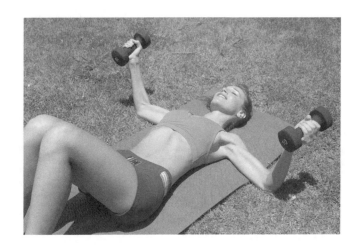

Naomi-type	8–12 reps
Demi-type	10–15 reps
Madonna-type	15–20 reps
Beginner	5-lb weight
Intermediate	10-lb weight
Advanced	15-lb weight

POSITION
- Lie on your back on a mat.
- Bend your knees and place your feet flat on the ground.
- Bend your elbows 90 degrees so that your elbows and triceps are resting on the ground, and extend them out away from your body, exposing your armpits.
- Your elbows should be at shoulder level.
- Hold the dumbbells with your palms facing each other.

MOVEMENT
- Engage your chest, arms, and back and lower the dumbbells to the ground until your arms are almost straight but still slightly bent.
- Do not let your hands touch the ground.
- Once you reach the bottom position, slowly and with control, raise your hands to the starting position.
- Repeat until you complete one set.

Up the Ante

Increase the Intensity

An exercise program needs to progress for continued benefits. To up the ante of a cardio program, increase the intensity at a controlled pace as opposed to suddenly going to an extreme and adding too much time, exertion, or distance. If your regular routine consists of walking, to intensify the exercise you can increase the duration and add a few extra minutes, or increase the exertion by intermittently adding a few minutes of jogging, incorporating stairs, or increasing the incline with hills. For a resistance routine, you can add intensity by increasing the weight or doing more reps.

Dumbbell Press with Twist

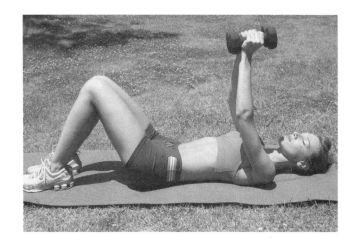

Naomi-type	8–12 reps
Demi-type	10–15 reps
Madonna-type	15–20 reps
Beginner	5-lb weight
Intermediate	10-lb weight
Advanced	15-lb weight

POSITION
- Lie on your back on a mat.
- Bend your knees and place your feet flat on the ground.
- Bend your elbows 90 degrees, folding your forearms back so that the tops of your hands fall on your shoulders.
- Your elbows should be at shoulder level with your elbows and triceps resting on the ground.
- Hold the dumbbells with your palms facing your hips.

MOVEMENT
- Engage your chest, arms, and back and press the dumbbells straight up above your chest while twisting your palms so that they are facing each other when your arms are fully extended.
- Press until your arms are straight, without locking your elbows.
- Once you reach the top position, slowly and with control, lower your hands to the starting position while twisting your palms back to the starting position.
- Be sure you lower your arms all the way down until your elbows and triceps are again resting on the ground.
- Repeat until you complete one set.

Dumbbell Press, Palms Facing Each Other

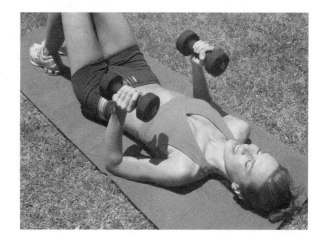

Naomi-type	8–12 reps
Demi-type	10–15 reps
Madonna-type	15–20 reps
Beginner	5-lb weight
Intermediate	10-lb weight
Advanced	15-lb weight

POSITION

- Lie on your back on a mat.
- Bend your knees and place your feet flat on the ground.
- Bend your elbows 90 degrees, folding your forearms back so that the tops of your hands fall on your shoulders.
- Your elbows should be at your sides against your ribs with your elbows and triceps resting on the ground.
- Hold the dumbbells with your palms facing each other.

MOVEMENT

- Engage your chest, arms, and back and press the dumbbells straight up above your chest, keeping your palms facing each other.
- Press until your arms are straight, without locking your elbows.
- Your dumbbells should be touching each other above your chest.
- Once you reach the top position, slowly and with control, lower your hands to the starting position.
- Be sure you lower your arms all the way down until your elbows and triceps are again resting on the ground.
- Repeat until you complete one set.

Standing Bicep Curl

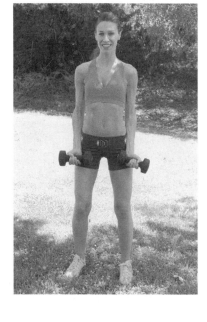

Naomi-type	6–8 reps
Demi-type	8–12 reps
Madonna-type	12–15 reps
Beginner	5-lb weight
Intermediate	10-lb weight
Advanced	15-lb weight

POSITION

- Stand up straight with your feet shoulder-width apart.
- Let your arms hang at your sides.
- Bend your knees slightly.
- Hold the dumbbells with your palms facing up.

MOVEMENT

- Keep your elbows and upper arms pressed against the sides of your rib cage as you bend your elbows and lift the dumbbells using your forearms.
- Your forearms are the only part of your body that will move.
- Keep your wrists strong and long. Do not let them bend.
- Lift the dumbbells toward your shoulders.
- Keep your palms up during the full range of motion.
- Squeeze your biceps at the top of the movement—this is the contraction.
- Slowly lower the dumbbells to the starting position.
- Repeat (this movement can be performed using both arms together or alternating arms) until you complete one set.

Up the Ante

Exercise Sitting Down

You might think that sitting down takes some of the edge off this exercise, but sitting on a stability ball actually adds extra oomph. When sitting on a stability ball you are forced to place focus on your arms as well as all your stabilizing muscles, which are keeping you from rolling off the ball.

Standing Bicep Curl with Twist

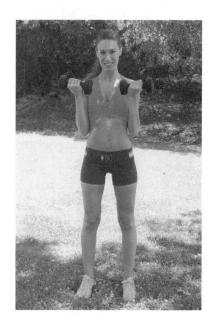

Naomi-type	6–8 reps
Demi-type	8–12 reps
Madonna-type	12–15 reps
Beginner	5-lb weight
Intermediate	10-lb weight
Advanced	15-lb weight

POSITION
- Stand up straight with your feet shoulder-width apart.
- Let your arms hang at your sides.
- Bend your knees slightly.
- Hold the dumbbells with your palms facing your hips.

MOVEMENT
- Keep your elbows and upper arms pressed against the sides of your rib cage as you bend your elbows and lift the dumbbells using your forearms.
- As you lift, twist your wrists outward.
- The twisting movement should require full range of motion from the initiation of the lift through the contraction at the top of the movement.
- Your forearms are the only part of your body that will move.
- Keep your wrists strong and long. Do not let them bend.
- Lift the dumbbells toward your shoulders.
- Squeeze your biceps at the top of the movement—this is the contraction.
- Slowly lower the dumbbells to the starting position as you twist your wrists inward.
- Repeat (this movement can be performed using both arms together or alternating arms) until you complete one set.

Sprint Curl

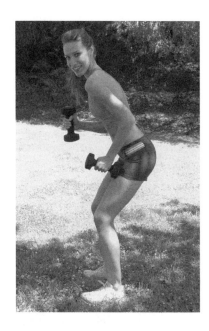

Naomi-type	6–8 reps
Demi-type	8–12 reps
Madonna-type	12–15 reps
Beginner	5-lb weight
Intermediate	10-lb weight
Advanced	15-lb weight

POSITION
- Stand straight with your feet shoulder-width apart.
- Bend your knees 45 degrees.
- Slightly bend your torso forward from your waist.
- Keep your back long and align your neck with your back.
- Hold the dumbbells with your palms facing your hips.
- Slightly bend your elbows and allow the dumbbells to lean on the sides of your quads.

MOVEMENT
- Keep your elbows and upper arms pressed against the sides of your rib cage as you bend your elbows and, using your forearms, lift one dumbbell up to your shoulder.
- Squeeze your biceps at the top of the movement—this is the contraction.
- As soon as you reach the top of the movement, begin to lower that dumbbell as you simultaneously lift the other dumbbell.
- Continue lifting alternating dumbbells in a constant flow.
- Your forearms are the only part of your body that will move.
- Keep your wrists strong and long. Do not let them bend.
- Repeat until you complete one set.

90-Degree Bicep Curl

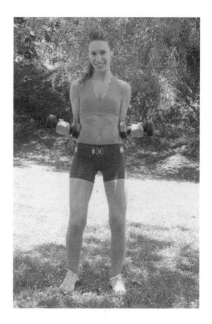

Naomi-type	6–8 reps
Demi-type	8–12 reps
Madonna-type	12–15 reps
Beginner	5-lb weight
Intermediate	10-lb weight
Advanced	15-lb weight

POSITION
- Stand straight with your feet shoulder-width apart.
- Let your arms hang at your sides.
- Bend your knees slightly.
- Hold the dumbbells with your palms facing up.
- Bend your elbows and curl your forearms up so that your elbows are bent 90 degrees.

MOVEMENT
- Keep your elbows and upper arms pressed against the sides of your rib cage as you lift the dumbbells to your shoulders.
- Your forearms are the only part of your body that will move.
- Keep your wrists strong and long. Do not let them bend.
- Squeeze your biceps at top of the movement—this is the contraction.
- Slowly lower the dumbbells to the starting position.
- Repeat (this movement can be performed using both arms together or alternating arms) until you complete one set.

Tricep Dip

Naomi-type	6–8 reps
Demi-type	8–12 reps
Madonna-type	12–15 reps

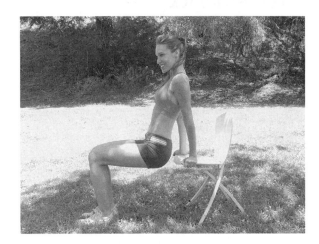

POSITION

- Sit on a sturdy chair or bench.
- Place your arms at your sides, your hands on the sides of the chair with your palms facing down and your fingers bending over the edges.
- Lift your butt up off the chair and support your body weight with your hands on the chair and your feet on the ground.
- Press your body forward so that your butt is no longer on the chair but is elevated just off the front of the chair. The back of your butt should be aligned with the seat of your chair.
- Your arms should be straight.
- Your knees should be bent 90 degrees.
- Keep your back long and straight.

MOVEMENT

- Slowly and with control, bend your elbows and lower your body toward the ground until your elbows are bent 90 degrees.
- Keep your back close to the chair to prevent anterior shoulder strain.
- Once your downward position is reached, use your triceps to push you back up to the starting position.
- Repeat until you complete one set.

Up the Ante

Tricep Dip Extra

To add a little extra to this movement, extend your legs out to a straight position so that your heels are the only part of your feet touching the ground. Too tough? Straighten just one leg. Another way is to elevate your legs on an opposing chair or bench. Just be sure not to push yourself beyond your capabilities. We are not aiming for injury, we are aiming to increase strength.

Tricep Kickback

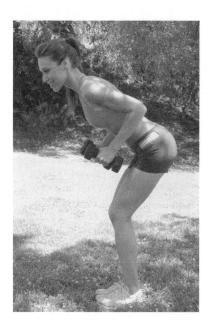

Naomi-type	6–8 reps
Demi-type	8–12 reps
Madonna-type	12–15 reps
Beginner	2-lb weight
Intermediate	5-lb weight
Advanced	8-lb weight

POSITION
- Stand straight with your feet shoulder-width apart.
- Bend forward 45 degrees at the waist.
- Hold the dumbbells with your palms facing your hips.
- Bend your elbows 90 degrees and press your elbows and upper arms against your rib cage.

MOVEMENT
- Keeping your elbows pressed against your rib cage, flex your arms straight behind you, straightening your elbows.
- Fully contract your triceps before slowly bending your elbows and lowering your forearms to the starting position.
- Repeat (this exercise can be performed using both arms together or alternating arms) until you complete one set.

Basic Crunch

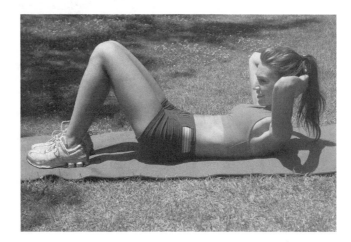

Naomi-type	25 reps
Demi-type	15 reps
Madonna-type	50 reps

POSITION
- Lie on your back on a mat.
- Bend your knees and place your feet flat on the ground a few inches below your butt.
- Bend your elbows and rest your hands behind your head (this is not a grip; you are just resting your hands).

MOVEMENT
- Exhale as you tighten your abs and lift your shoulder blades off the ground (remember, your hands are just resting; do not let your arms push you off the ground).
- Do not pull through your neck. Keep your neck straight from your spine to the top of your head. The only reason your hands are there is to support your head and release the strain from your neck. This exercise targets your abs, not your neck or arms.
- Keep your lower back flat on the ground. You will not sit up completely.
- Once you have come up as far as you can without lifting your lower back off the ground, slowly and with control, lower your upper back, shoulder blades, and head down to the ground.
- Repeat until you complete one set.

Crunch with Feet Up

Naomi-type	25 reps
Demi-type	15 reps
Madonna-type	50 reps

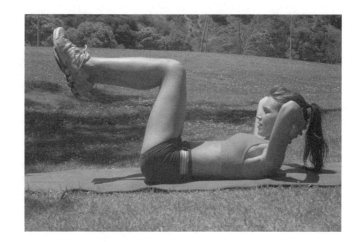

POSITION

- Lie on your back on a mat.
- Bend your knees and lift your feet up off the ground so that your knees are bent 90 degrees and there is a 90-degree bend at your hips.
- Bend your elbows and rest your hands behind your head (this is not a grip; you are just resting your hands).

MOVEMENT

- Exhale as you tighten your abs and lift your shoulder blades off the ground (remember, your hands are just resting; do not let your arms push you off the ground).
- Do not pull through your neck. Keep your neck straight from your spine to the top of your head. The only reason your hands are there is to support your head and release the strain from your neck. This exercise targets your abs, not your neck or arms.
- Keep your lower back flat along the ground. You will not sit up completely.
- Once you have come up as far as you can without lifting your lower back off the ground, slowly and with control, lower your upper back, shoulder blades, and head down to the ground.
- Repeat until you complete one set.

Reverse Ab Crunch

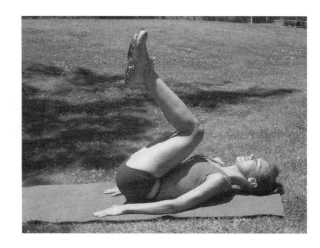

Naomi-type	25 reps
Demi-type	15 reps
Madonna-type	50 reps

POSITION

- Lie on your back on a mat.
- Bend your knees and lift your feet up off the ground so that your knees are bent 90 degrees and there is a 90-degree bend at your hips.
- Allow your arms to fall straight alongside your body.

MOVEMENT

- Exhale as you tighten your abs and lift your hips, butt, and lower back off the ground.
- Your knees will move toward your chest.
- Keep your upper back flat on the ground.
- Hold in that elevated position for 5 to 10 seconds.
- Slowly and with control, roll your hips, butt, and lower back down to the ground.
- Repeat until you complete one set.

Elbows to Knees, Knees to Elbows

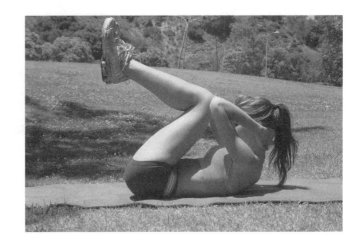

Naomi-type	25 reps
Demi-type	15 reps
Madonna-type	50 reps

POSITION

- Lie on your back on a mat.
- Bend your knees and place your feet flat on the ground a few inches below your butt.
- Bend your elbows and rest your hands behind your head (this is not a grip; you are just resting your hands).

MOVEMENT

- Exhale as you tighten your abs and lift your feet, hips, butt, and lower back off the ground. Your knees will move toward your chest.
- Tighten your abs again and raise your shoulder blades and upper back off the ground toward your elevated abs and legs.
- Your elbows and knees should be moving toward each other.
- Do not pull through your neck. Keep your neck straight from your spine to the top of your head. The only reason your hands are there is to support your head and release the strain from your neck. This exercise targets your abs, not your neck or arms.
- Hold this position, then slowly and with control, lower down to the ground.
- Repeat until you complete one set.

Modified Bicycle

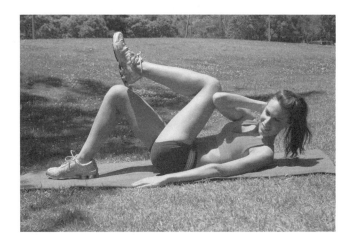

Naomi-type	25 reps
Demi-type	15 reps
Madonna-type	50 reps

POSITION
- Lie on your back on a mat.
- Bend your knees and place your feet flat on the ground.
- Bend your elbows and place your hands behind head, or bend one elbow and place that hand behind your head and extend the other arm flat along-side you. (Remember, your hands are there only to support your head, not to hoist you up. This exercise targets your abs, not your neck or arms.)

MOVEMENT
- Tighten your abs, exhale, and raise your shoulder blades off the ground.
- While maintaining the lifted position, twist your torso slightly to the left and focus on pulling your right elbow up to your left knee.
- Simultaneously raise your left foot off the ground and pull your left knee in toward your chest and your right elbow.
- Your right elbow and left knee should touch.
- Lower yourself back to the starting position with your knees bent, your feet flat on the ground, and your back on the ground.
- Repeat the movement on the opposite side.
- Alternate between the two sides until you complete one set.

Squat

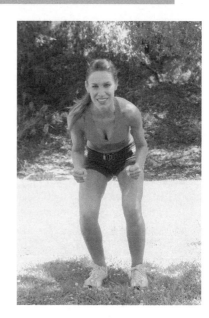

Naomi-type	10–15 reps
Demi-type	15–20 reps
Madonna-type	20–25 reps

POSITION

- Stand with your feet hip-width apart, toes facing forward.

MOVEMENT

- Slowly and with control, bend your knees to a 90-degree angle.
- Keep your knees over your toes by angling your knees slightly out as opposed to bending straight down.
- Be sure to maintain a straight back; don't hunch forward or lean backward.
- If you can't keep your heels on the ground, it is okay to raise them slightly.
- Hold for a just a second in that lowered position, then slowly raise your body, straightening your legs to the original position.
- As you straighten your knees, focus on putting some of the energy into your glutes, engaging them as you stand.
- Repeat until you complete one set.

Plié Squat

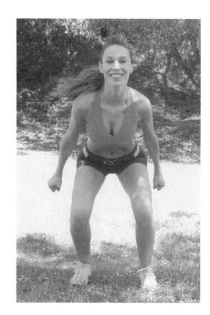

Naomi-type	10–15 reps
Demi-type	15–20 reps
Madonna-type	20–25 reps

POSITION

- Stand with your feet hip-width apart, then separate them an additional 6 to 12 inches.
- Slightly angle your toes out and your heels in at a 45-degree angle.

MOVEMENT

- Slowly and with control, bend your knees to a 90-degree angle.
- Keep your knees over your toes by angling your knees slightly out as opposed to bending straight down.
- Your center of balance will fall between your feet.
- Be sure to maintain a straight back; don't hunch forward or lean backward.
- If you can't keep your heels on the ground, it is okay to raise them slightly.
- Hold for a just a second in that lowered position, then slowly raise your body, straightening your legs to the original position.
- As you straighten your knees, focus on putting some of the energy into your glutes, engaging them as you stand.
- Repeat until you complete one set.

Ski Squat

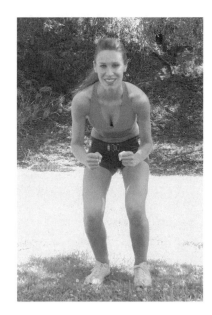

Naomi-type	10–15 reps
Demi-type	15–20 reps
Madonna-type	20–25 reps

POSITION
- Stand with your feet hip-width apart, toes facing forward.

MOVEMENT
- Slowly and with control, bend your knees to a 90-degree angle.
- Keep your knees over your toes by angling your knees slightly out as opposed to bending straight down.
- Be sure to maintain a straight back; don't hunch forward or lean backward.
- If you can't keep your heels on the ground, it is okay to raise them slightly.
- Hold in this lowered position for a second.
- Slowly raise your body 4 to 6 inches. Do not straighten your legs completely. Those 4 to 6 inches are your full range of motion.
- As you straighten your knees, focus on putting some of the energy into your glutes, engaging them as you stand.
- Repeat until you complete one set.

Frog Squat

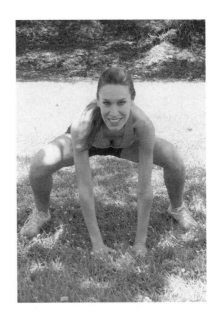

Naomi-type	10–15 reps
Demi-type	15–20 reps
Madonna-type	20–25 reps

POSITION

- Stand with your feet hip-width apart, then separate them an additional 6 to 12 inches.
- Slightly angle your toes out and your heels in at a 45-degree angle.
- Keeping your legs as straight as you can, bend forward at your waist until you can touch your fingers to the ground.

MOVEMENT

- Slowly and with control, bend your knees, lowering your glutes until your knees are bent 90 degrees.
- Keep your arms straight.
- Keep your knees over your toes by angling your knees slightly out as opposed to bending straight down.
- Hold in this lowered position for a second.
- Slowly push through your quads to straighten your legs, keeping your hands on the ground.
- Repeat until you complete one set.

Alternate Lunge

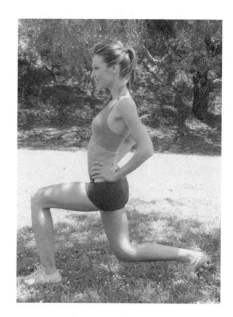

Naomi-type	10—15 reps
Demi-type	15—20 reps
Madonna-type	20—25 reps

POSITION
- Stand with your feet hip-width apart, toes facing forward.

MOVEMENT
- Step one leg forward about 2 feet.
- You should land the forward moving leg on the ball of your foot, then roll through your foot, placing the entire foot on the ground.
- As you land, both knees will bend 90 degrees so that the knee of the back standing leg is almost touching the ground and the quad of the front leg is parallel to the ground.
- Your back heel should be raised slightly off the ground, with the majority of your weight on the ball of the foot.
- Your feet should still be hip-width apart. You don't want one foot to be right in front of the other.
- Engage your quads and the glute of your standing back leg as you propel your front leg back to the starting standing position.
- Repeat the same motion on the opposite leg.
- Continue with the repetitions, switching your legs back and forth until you complete one set.

Single-Leg Lunge

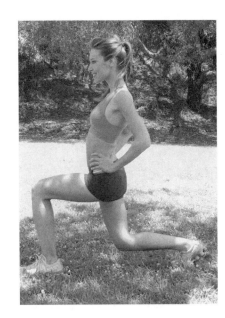

Naomi-type	10–15 reps
Demi-type	15–20 reps
Madonna-type	20–25 reps

POSITION

- Stand with your feet hip-width apart, toes facing forward.

MOVEMENT

- Step one leg forward about 2 feet.
- You should land the forward moving leg on the ball of your foot, then roll through your foot, placing the entire foot on the ground.
- As you land, both knees will bend 90 degrees so that the knee of the back standing leg is almost touching the ground and the quad of the front leg is parallel to the ground.
- Your back heel should be raised slightly off the ground, with the majority of weight on the ball of the foot.
- Your feet should still be hip-width apart. You don't want one foot to be right in front of the other.
- Engage your quads and the glute of your standing back leg as you propel your front leg back to the starting standing position.
- Repeat on the same leg.
- After completing one set, switch to the opposite leg.

Pump Lunge

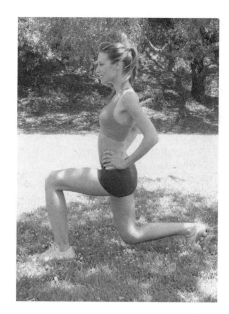

Naomi-type	10–15 reps
Demi-type	15–20 reps
Madonna-type	20–25 reps

POSITION
- Stand with your feet hip-width apart, toes facing forward.

MOVEMENT
- Step one leg forward about 2 feet.
- Land the forward-moving leg on the ball of your foot, then roll through your foot, placing the entire foot on the ground.
- As you land, both knees will bend 90 degrees so that the knee of the back standing leg is almost touching the ground and the quad of the front leg is parallel to the ground.
- Your back heel should be raised slightly off the ground, with the majority of your weight on the ball of the foot.
- Your feet should still be hip-width apart. You don't want one foot to be right in front of the other.
- Hold this position for 5 to 10 seconds.
- Engage your quads and the glute of your standing back leg as you slowly raise your legs 4 to 6 inches without completely straightening your knees.
- Once that position has been reached, return your knees to the 90-degree bent position. This is a slow and controlled pumping motion.
- Repeat the pump until one set is complete.
- Engage your quads and the glute of your standing back leg as you propel your front leg back to the starting standing position.
- After completing one set, switch to the opposite leg.

Russian Lunge

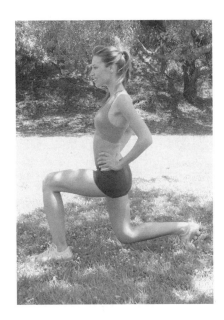

Naomi-type	10–15 reps
Demi-type	15–20 reps
Madonna-type	20–25 reps

POSITION
- Stand with your feet hip-width apart, toes facing forward.

MOVEMENT
- Step one leg forward about 2 feet.
- Land the forward-moving leg on the ball of your foot, then roll through your foot, placing the entire foot on the ground.
- As you land, both knees will bend 90 degrees so that the knee of the back standing leg is almost touching the ground and the quad of the front leg is parallel to the ground.
- Your back heel should be raised slightly off the ground, with the majority of your weight on the ball of the foot.
- Your feet should still be hip-width apart. You don't want one foot to be right in front of the other.
- Engage your quads and the glute of your standing back leg and power into a jump straight up into the air.
- While in midair, switch leg positions so that you land with the opposite leg forward and the opposite leg back. Be sure to land with your knees bent in order to avoid injury.
- Repeat back and forth until you complete one set.

Single-Leg Chair Lunge

Naomi-type	10–15 reps
Demi-type	15–20 reps
Madonna-type	20–25 reps

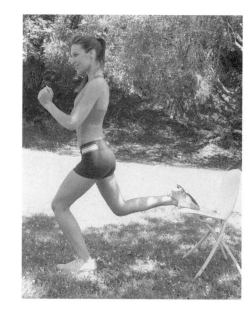

POSITION
- Stand 2 to 3 feet from a sturdy chair, step, or bench, with your back to it.
- Place one foot on top of the chair behind you (keep your front standing leg straight).
- Be sure to maintain hip-width distance between your legs.
- Let your arms hang at your sides.

MOVEMENT
- Slowly and with control, bend the knee of your standing leg 90 degrees.
- Your knee should not push past your toe. If it does, you need to readjust your front foot placement. Your knee should be over your toe in the bent position.
- Be sure to keep your back straight.
- Your back elevated leg should maintain a slight bend.
- Once you have bent into the downward position, use the quad and glute of your front leg to power yourself back up to the starting standing position.
- In order to really work the quad, push up through the ball of your front foot.
- After completing one set, switch to the opposite leg.

Alternate Step-Up

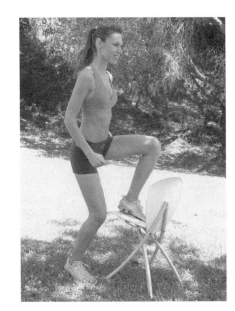

Naomi-type	10–15 reps
Demi-type	15–20 reps
Madonna-type	20–25 reps

POSITION
- Stand straight facing a sturdy chair, step, or bench.
- Let your arms hang at your sides.

MOVEMENT
- Step up onto the chair with one leg, placing your entire foot on the chair, and propel yourself up so that all your weight is placed on that front foot.
- Straighten both legs.
- Your back leg will rise off the ground.
- Once you reach the fully elevated position, bend your front supporting leg, allowing your back leg to begin to lower to the ground.
- Once your back leg touches the ground, bring your front leg down to meet it.
- Continue with the repetitions, switching your legs back and forth until you complete one set.

Single-Leg Step-Up

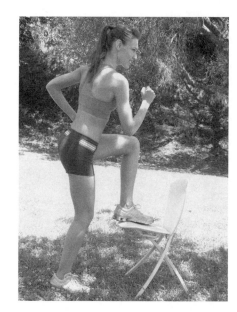

Naomi-type	10–15 reps
Demi-type	15–20 reps
Madonna-type	20–25 reps

POSITION
- Stand straight facing a sturdy chair, step, or bench.
- Let your arms hang at your sides.

MOVEMENT
- Step up onto the chair with one leg, placing your entire foot on the chair, and propel yourself up so that all your weight is placed on that front foot.
- Straighten both legs.
- Your back leg will rise off the ground.
- Once you reach the fully elevated position, bend your front supporting leg, allowing your back leg to begin to lower to the ground.
- Once your back leg touches the ground, keep the front leg up on the chair and repeat the motion with the same leg.
- Focus on the quad of your front leg to propel your body up and carefully return your back leg back down to the ground with a slightly bent knee to cushion the impact.
- To increase your heart rate, include your arms in the motion by moving them back and forth as you would when running.
- Repeat until you complete one set.

Wall Sit

Naomi-type	45 seconds
Demi-type	30 seconds
Madonna-type	60 seconds

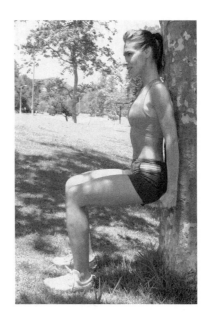

POSITION
- Stand 1½ to 2 feet away from a wall.
- Your feet should be hip-width apart.
- Bend your knees 90 degrees and allow your back to push up against the wall.
- You are in a sitting position, except that there is no chair to support you. The support is the force of your torso pushing against the wall.

MOVEMENT
- Hold this position.
- Maintain the distance between your knees—do not let them touch.
- Take deep belly breaths to get through it.
- Be sure that your entire back is pushing against the wall without any arch in your lower back.
- Flex your abs and pull them in toward your spine.
- Press through the balls of your feet to further push your body against the wall.
- Finally, release and stand up.

Wall Sit with Inner-Thigh Squeeze

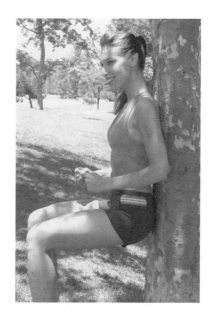

Naomi-type	45 seconds
Demi-type	30 seconds
Madonna-type	60 seconds

POSITION
- Stand 1½ to 2 feet away from a wall.
- Place your feet together.
- Bend your knees 90 degrees and allow your back to push up against the wall.
- You are in a sitting position, except that there is no chair to support you. The support is the force of your torso pushing against the wall.

MOVEMENT
- Hold this position.
- Press your knees and thighs against each other.
- Take deep belly breaths to get through it.
- Be sure that your entire back is pushing against the wall without any arch in your lower back.
- Flex your abs and pull them in toward your spine.
- Press through the balls of your feet to further push your body against the wall.
- Keep squeezing your knees and thighs together.
- Finally, release and stand up.

Power Skating

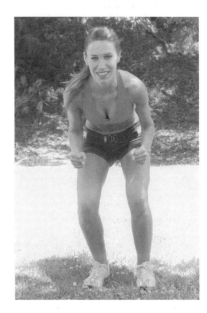

Naomi-type	10–15 reps
Demi-type	Skip this exercise
Madonna-type	40–50 reps

POSITION

- Stand with your feet hip-width apart, toes facing forward.
- Slightly bend forward at your waist.
- Let your arms hang at your sides.

MOVEMENT

- You will be moving in a side-to-side motion, with the goal of creating a distance of 4 feet between each standing position.
- Lift your right foot about 1 inch off the ground.
- Create force in the inner edge of your left foot as you drive your right leg out to the side, skimming the ground and landing on that leg approximately 4 feet away.
- For a moment your legs will be wide apart, until you lift the left leg off the ground and set it down at the right leg. Keep the feet hip-width apart.
- You can use your arms to help create force by swinging them from side to side in conjunction with your leg movements.
- Repeat this motion moving in the opposite direction, returning to the starting position.
- Continue to do this low leap back and forth until you complete one set.

Bunny Hop

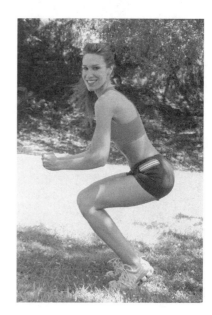

Naomi-type	10–15 reps
Demi-type	Skip this exercise
Madonna-type	40–50 reps

POSITION
- Stand with your feet hip-width apart, toes facing forward.
- Bend your knees to 45 degrees.
- Allow your torso to slightly bend forward from your waist.
- Your knees should be slightly past your toes to protect your knees.
- Keep the balls of your feet on the ground and your heels slightly elevated.

MOVEMENT
- Maintain your body position and slowly and with control, push up off your toes.
- Your toes will rise off the ground.
- Repeat this motion while increasing the tempo of the hop so that you are moving up and down faster and faster.
- Repeat until you complete one set.

Jump Lunge

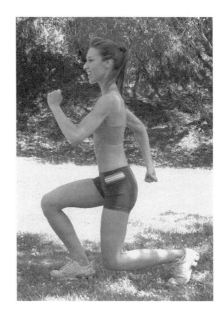

Naomi-type	8–12 reps
Demi-type	Skip this exercise
Madonna-type	20–25 reps

POSITION

- Stand with your feet hip-width apart, toes facing forward.
- Step one leg forward about 2 feet.
- Land the forward-moving leg on the ball of your foot, then roll through your foot, placing the entire foot on the ground.
- As you land, both knees will bend 90 degrees so that the knee of the back standing leg is almost touching the ground and the quad of the front leg is parallel to the ground.
- Your back heel should be raised slightly off the ground, with the majority of your weight on the ball of the foot.

MOVEMENT

- Engage your quads and the glute of your standing back leg as you propel your body straight up into the air.
- Your legs will straighten in the air.
- As you fall back into the starting position, bend your knees to cushion your landing.
- Let the balls of your feet touch the ground first, then allow the front foot to roll to a fully flat position.
- Return your knees to the bent 90-degree position.
- Repeat on the same leg.
- After completing one set, switch to the opposite leg.

4-Count Jump Lunge

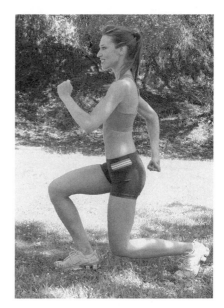

Naomi-type	8–12 reps
Demi-type	Skip this exercise
Madonna-type	25–30 reps

POSITION
- Stand with your feet hip-width apart, toes facing forward.
- Step one leg forward about 2 feet.
- Land the forward-moving leg on the ball of your foot, then roll through your foot, placing the entire foot on the ground.
- As you land, both knees will bend 90 degrees so that the knee of the back standing leg is almost touching the ground and the quad of the front leg is parallel to the ground.
- Your back heel should be raised slightly off the ground, with the majority of your weight on the ball of the foot.

MOVEMENT
- While in the lunge position, raise your knees 4 to 6 inches without fully straightening your legs.
- Return your knees to the bent 90-degree position.
- Repeat this 3 more times so that you are pumping your legs up and down.
- After your fourth pump, engage your quads and the glute of your standing back leg as you propel your body straight up into the air.
- Your legs will straighten in the air.
- As you fall back into the starting position, bend your knees to cushion your landing.
- Let the balls of your feet touch the ground first, then allow the front foot to roll to a fully flat position.
- Return your knees to the bent 90-degree position.
- Repeat on the same leg.
- After completing one set, switch to the opposite leg.

Alternating Jump Lunge

Naomi-type	10–15 reps
Demi-type	Skip this exercise
Madonna-type	20–25 reps

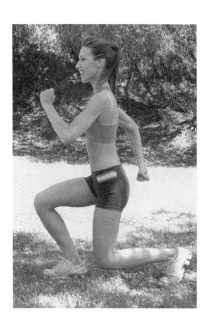

For instructions, see the Russian Lunge on page 165.

Jump Squat

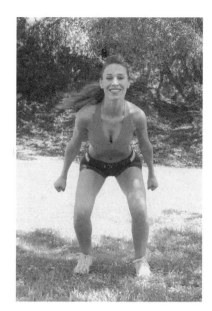

Naomi-type	8–12 reps
Demi-type	Skip this exercise
Madonna-type	20–25 reps

POSITION
- Stand with your feet hip-width apart, toes facing forward, arms at your sides.
- Bend your knees 45 degrees.
- Keep your back straight.
- Allow your arms to bend at the elbow.

MOVEMENT
- Slowly and with control, bend your knees to a 90-degree angle.
- Keep your knees over your toes by angling your knees slightly out as opposed to bending straight down.
- If you can't keep your heels on the ground, it is okay to raise them slightly.
- Pull your arms back.
- Propel your body up and forward, throwing your arms forward to further create the thrust.
- The goal is to see how far you can jump without losing your balance.
- Be sure to land with bent knees.
- Hold in that 90-degree bent-knee position for a few seconds.
- Once you have gained your balance, stand up to the starting 45-degree bent-knee position.
- Repeat, moving forward, until you have completed one set.

4-Count Jump Squat

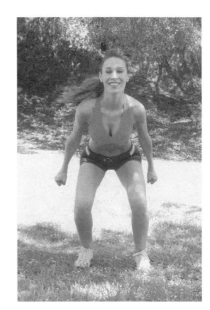

Naomi-type	8–12 reps
Demi-type	Skip this exercise
Madonna-type	25–30 reps

POSITION
- Stand with your feet hip-width apart, toes facing forward, arms at your sides.
- Bend your knees 45 degrees.
- Keep your back straight.
- Allow your arms to bend at the elbow.

MOVEMENT
- Slowly and with control, bend your knees to a 90-degree angle.
- Keep your knees over your toes by angling your knees slightly out as opposed to bending straight down.
- If you can't keep your heels on the ground, it is okay to raise them slightly.
- Pull your arms back.
- Raise your knees 4 to 6 inches, without completely straightening your legs.
- Return to the 90-degree bent-knee position.
- Repeat this 3 more times, pumping your legs up and down.
- Return to the 90-degree bent-knee position.
- Propel your body up and forward, throwing your arms forward to further create the thrust.
- The goal is to see how far you can jump without losing your balance.
- Be sure to land with bent knees.
- Hold in that 90-degree bent-knee position for a few seconds.
- Once you have gained your balance, stand up to the starting 45-degree bent-knee position.
- Repeat, moving forward, until you complete one set.

Leg Extension

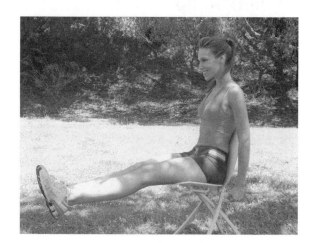

Naomi-type	8–12 reps
Demi-type	15–20 reps
Madonna-type	20–25 reps

POSITION
- Sit upright in a chair.
- Keep your back long and straight, your head tall.
- Your knees should be bent 90 degrees, with your feet placed on the ground.

MOVEMENT
- Focus on your quads as you extend your legs up, straightening your knees so that your legs are at a 90-degree angle to your torso.
- Slowly and with control, bend your knees back down so that your feet return to the ground.
- Repeat until you complete one set.

Single-Leg Extension

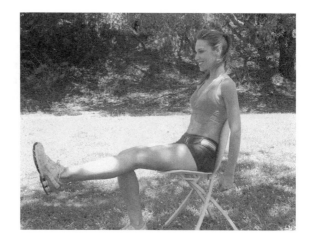

Naomi-type	8–12 reps
Demi-type	15–20 reps
Madonna-type	20–25 reps

POSITION
- Sit upright in a chair.
- Keep your back long and straight, your head tall.
- Your knees should be bent 90 degrees, with your feet flat on the ground.

MOVEMENT
- Focus on your quads as you extend one leg up, straightening your knee so that your elevated leg is at a 90-degree angle to your torso.
- Slowly and with control, bend your knee back down so that your foot falls flat on the ground next to your other foot.
- Repeat until you complete one set. Switch legs and repeat.

30-Degree Leg Extension

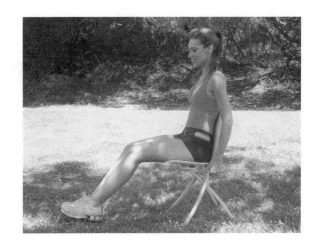

Naomi-type	8–12 reps
Demi-type	15–20 reps
Madonna-type	30–35 reps

POSITION
- Sit upright in a chair.
- Keep your back long and straight, your head tall.
- Your knees should be bent 90 degrees, with your feet flat on the ground.

MOVEMENT
- Focus on your quads as you extend your legs 5 inches off the ground.
- Your legs should be extended out from your body on a downward angle. Don't let your knees roll out to either side.
- Your toes should barely be raised off the ground.
- Slowly and with control, bend your knees back down so that your feet are flat on the ground.
- Repeat in a pumping motion until you complete one set.

Isometric Leg Extension

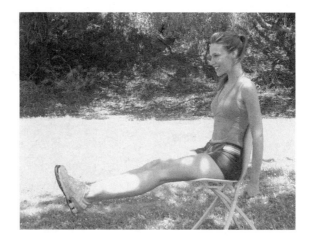

Naomi-type Demi-type Madonna-type	The length of the hold is the same for all three body types.

POSITION
- Sit upright in a chair.
- Keep your back long and straight, your head tall.
- Your knees should be bent at 90 degrees, with your feet flat on the ground.

MOVEMENT
- Focus on your quads as you extend your legs up, straightening your knees so that your legs are at a 90-degree angle to your torso.
- Hold your legs in the extended position for 30 seconds.
- Slowly and with control, bend your knees back down so that your feet fall flat on the ground.
- Repeat, but this time hold your legs elevated for 45 seconds.
- Repeat, but this time hold your legs elevated for 60 seconds.

Single-Leg Curl

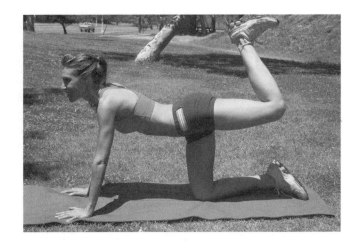

Naomi-type	8–12 reps
Demi-type	15–20 reps
Madonna-type	20–25 reps

POSITION

- On a mat, form a bridge with your body so that your weight is distributed equally between your hands and knees, with your stomach facing the ground.
- Keep your back flat and your head up—do not bend your neck down.
- Extend one leg straight back with your knee in a locked position so that your elevated leg is parallel to the ground.
- Be sure that your back remains level, creating a straight line along your back through your extended leg.

MOVEMENT

- Flex the knee of your elevated leg to bring your foot up to your glute.
- You will be working your hamstring and glute.
- Return to the starting elevated and extended-straight-leg position.
- Repeat with the same leg until you have completed one set.
- Switch legs and repeat.

Leg Curl

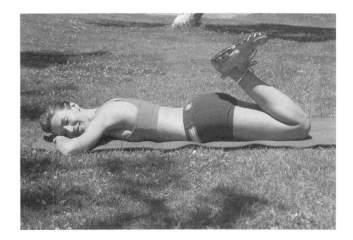

POSITION
- Lie flat on your stomach on a mat with your legs extended straight and together behind you.
- Be sure that your hips are pressing down into the ground.

MOVEMENT
- Bend and flex both knees to bring your feet up to your glutes.
- You will be working your hamstrings and glutes.
- Return to the starting position, resting your legs on the ground.
- Repeat until you complete one set.

Straight-Leg Lift

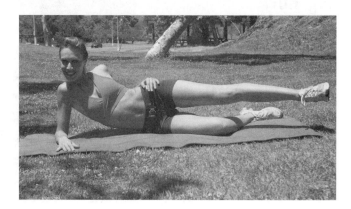

Naomi-type	10–15 reps
Demi-type	20–25 reps
Madonna-type	35–50 reps

POSITION
- Lie on one side on a mat.
- Your legs should be stacked on top of each other. Bend your lower arm to a 45-degree angle and lean on it to support your upper body. Rest your other arm on your hip. Keep your head lifted and straight.
- Bend the bottom knee (the one touching the ground) so that your leg is at a 45-degree angle.
- Keep your top leg straight and flex the foot.
- Keep your hips stacked straight up and down.

MOVEMENT
- Keep your top leg straight as you lift it up a few inches until the heel is level with the top of your hip.
- Lower your leg back down to the starting position.
- Repeat until you complete one set.
- Switch legs and repeat.

45-Degree Leg Lift

Naomi-type	10–15 reps
Demi-type	20–25 reps
Madonna-type	35–50 reps

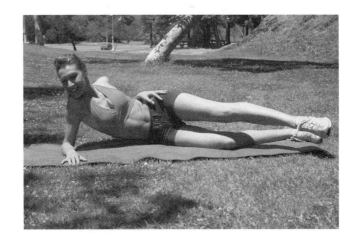

POSITION

- Lie on one side on a mat.
- Your legs should be stacked on top of each other. Bend your lower arm to a 45-degree angle and lean on it to support your upper body. Rest your other arm on your hip. Keep your head lifted and straight.
- Bend both knees so that your legs are at a 45-degree angle.
- Bend forward at your waist 45 degrees.
- Your legs should remain stacked in the same position on top of each other.
- Straighten your top leg.
- Flex both feet.
- Keep your hips stacked straight up and down.

MOVEMENT

- Lift your top leg, raising it 5 inches.
- Be sure that your knee and foot move together so that they are constantly at the same height.
- Lower your leg back down to the starting position.
- Repeat until you complete one set.
- Switch legs and repeat.

90-Degree Leg Lift

Naomi-type	10–15 reps
Demi-type	20–25 reps
Madonna-type	35–50 reps

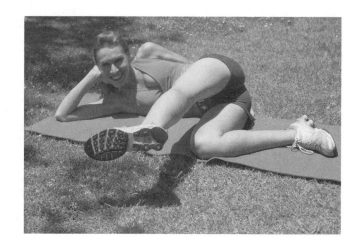

POSITION
- Lie on one side on a mat.
- Your legs should be stacked on top of each other. Bend your lower arm to a 45-degree angle and lean on it to support your upper body. Rest your other arm on your hip. Keep your head lifted and straight.
- Bend the bottom knee (the one touching the ground) so that your leg is at a 90-degree angle.
- Keep your upper body straight and move your top leg out in front of you so that it is at a 90-degree angle at your waist.
- Your legs should be stacked in the same position on top of each other.
- Keep your top leg straight.
- Flex both feet.
- Keep your hips stacked straight up and down.

MOVEMENT
- Lift your top leg, raising it to a vertical position so that the bottom of the foot faces up and the leg is 90 degrees to the body.
- Lower your leg back down to the starting position.
- Repeat until you complete one set.
- Switch legs and repeat.

45-Degree Circle

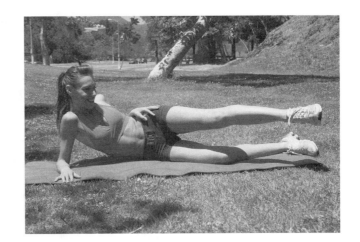

Naomi-type	10–15 reps
Demi-type	20–25 reps
Madonna-type	25–30 reps

POSITION
- Lie on one side on a mat.
- Your legs should be stacked on top of each other. Bend your lower arm to a 45-degree angle and lean on it to support your upper body. Rest your other arm on your hip. Keep your head lifted and straight.
- Bend forward at your waist 45 degrees.
- Bend the knee of your bottom leg 45 degrees.
- Keep your top leg straight.
- Flex both feet.
- Keep your hips stacked straight up and down.

MOVEMENT
- Lift your top leg 5 inches.
- Slowly and with control, rotate your top leg forward in a circular motion. The movement should come from the hip.
- Your circles should be at least 12 inches wide.
- Repeat in the same direction (forward) until you complete one set. Then change direction and repeat until you complete another set.
- Switch legs and repeat.

Lateral Leg Lift, Hands/Knees

Naomi-type	10–15 reps
Demi-type	20–25 reps
Madonna-type	35–50 reps

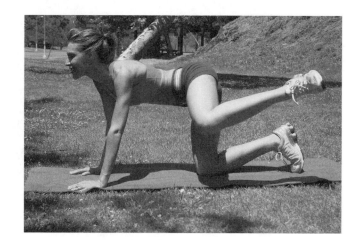

POSITION
- On a mat, form a bridge with your body so that your weight is distributed equally between your hands and knees, with your stomach facing the ground.
- Keep your back flat and your head up—do not bend your neck down.
- Flex the foot of your left leg.

MOVEMENT
- Keep the knee of your left leg bent as you raise it out to the side. The movement should come from the hip. Nothing else should move.
- Raise your leg 45 degrees off the ground.
- Slowly lower the knee back down to the ground, returning to your starting position.
- Repeat until you complete one set.
- Switch legs and repeat.

Glute Raise

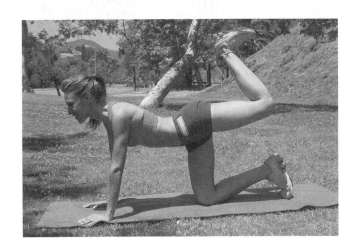

Naomi-type	10–15 reps
Demi-type	20–25 reps
Madonna-type	35–50 reps

POSITION
- On a mat, form a bridge with your body so that your weight is distributed equally between your hands and knees, with your stomach facing the ground.
- Keep your back flat and your head up—do not bend your neck down.
- Flex the foot of your left leg.

MOVEMENT
- Keep the knee of your left leg bent as you raise it back. The movement should come from the hip. Nothing else should move.
- Raise your leg 90 degrees off the ground, so that your quad is parallel to the ground.
- Engage your glutes to move your leg up and down.
- Slowly lower the knee back down to the ground, returning to your starting position.
- Repeat until you complete one set.
- Switch legs and repeat.

Tight Glute Raise

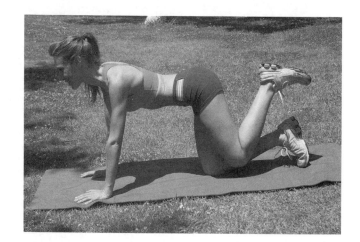

Naomi-type	10–15 reps
Demi-type	20–25 reps
Madonna-type	35–50 reps

POSITION
- On a mat, form a bridge with your body so that your weight is distributed equally between your hands and knees, with your stomach facing the ground
- Keep your back flat and your head up—do not bend your neck down.
- Flex the foot of your left leg.

MOVEMENT
- Keep the knee of your left leg bent as you raise it back. The movement should come from the hip. Nothing else should move.
- Raise your leg 90 degrees off the ground, so that your quad is parallel to the ground.
- Engage your glutes to move your leg up and down.
- Slowly lower the knee 2 to 4 inches.
- Raise the quad back up to the position parallel to the ground.
- Repeat until you complete one set.
- Slowly and with control, lower your knee to the ground, returning to your starting position.
- Switch legs and repeat.

Pelvic Thrust

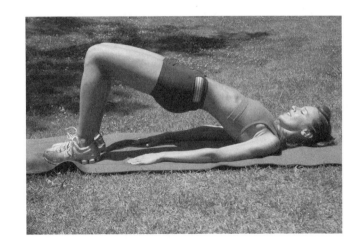

Naomi-type	10–15 reps
Demi-type	20–25 reps
Madonna-type	35–50 reps

POSITION
- Lie on your back on a mat.
- Bend your knees and place your feet flat on the ground.
- Your legs—from your feet to your knees—should be shoulder-width apart.
- Let your arms rest on the ground at your sides.

MOVEMENT
- Engage your glutes and raise your pelvis up off the ground. Your feet, upper back, and the back of your head will support your body weight.
- Lift your pelvis up until it forms a straight line from the top of your knees to your chest.
- Slowly lower your pelvis back down to the ground.
- Repeat until you complete one set.

Single-Leg Pelvic Thrust

Naomi-type	10–15 reps
Demi-type	20–25 reps
Madonna-type	35–50 reps

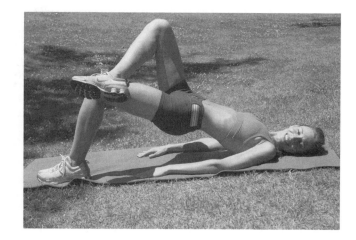

POSITION

- Lie on your back on a mat.
- Bend your knees and place your feet flat on the ground.
- Your legs—from your feet to your knees—should be shoulder-width apart.
- Let your arms rest on the ground at your sides.
- Cross your right leg over your left leg at the knee. Let your right calf hang down beside your left calf.

MOVEMENT

- Engage your glutes and raise your pelvis up off the ground. The foot of your left leg, your upper back, and the back of your head will support your body weight.
- Lift your pelvis up until it forms a straight line from the top of your knees to your chest.
- Slowly lower your pelvis back down to the ground.
- Repeat until you complete one set.

Pelvic Thrust Inner-Thigh Squeeze

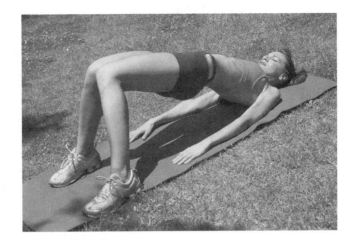

Naomi-type	10–15 reps
Demi-type	20–25 reps
Madonna-type	35–50 reps

POSITION
- Lie on your back on a mat.
- Bend your knees and place your feet flat on the ground.
- Press your knees and thighs together. Keep your feet separated.
- Let your arms rest on the ground at your sides.

MOVEMENT
- Squeeze your knees together and hold the squeeze through the entire set.
- Engage your glutes and raise your pelvis up off the ground. Your feet, upper back, and the back of your head will support your body weight.
- Lift your pelvis up until it forms a straight line from the top of your knees to your chest.
- Slowly lower your pelvis back down to the ground.
- Repeat until you complete one set.

On-Your-Back Hamstring Stretch

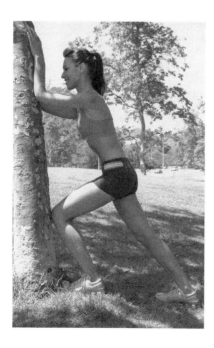

Works the hamstrings

- Lie on your back on a mat.
- Bend your knees and place your feet flat on the ground.
- Bring one knee to your chest, then stretch your leg straight up.
- Grasp your hands around the leg just under your knee.
- Gently pull your leg toward your face, trying to avoid bending your knee.
- If you must bend your knee, you can. Just be sure to maintain the stretch in the hamstring.
- Take 10 deep breaths.
- Switch legs and repeat.

Lunge Stretch

Works the hips and calves

- Stand facing a tree or another sturdy, tall, unmovable object.
- Bring both arms up and press your forearms against the support so that your triceps are parallel with the ground.
- Slide one leg straight back into a lunge position—this will force your front knee to bend to a 90-degree angle.
- Roll your tailbone under, keep your abs tights, and gently push your back heel down to create a stretch.
- Take 10 deep breaths.
- Switch legs and repeat.

Knees to Chest

Works the lower back and butt

- Lie on your back on a mat.
- Bend your knees and bring your thighs to your chest.
- Let your calves fall onto your hamstrings.
- Slightly separate your knees.
- Hold the back of your legs with your hands.
- Gently pull your knees closer to your chest until your butt slightly lifts from the ground.
- Keep your upper body relaxed.
- Take 10 deep breaths.

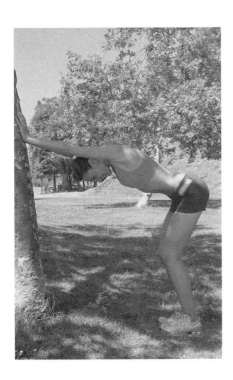

Back Stretch

Works the entire back, the shoulders, and the back of the neck

- Stand with your feet hip-width apart, 2 to 3 feet away from a tree or another sturdy, tall, unmovable object.
- Bend forward from your waist, then reach out and press both hands against the support, your arms outstretched.
- Slightly bend your knees and, keeping your grasp tight, flex and pull your back away from the support.
- Let your head drop gently forward until you feel the stretch from your neck all the way down your spine.
- Take 10 deep breaths.

9

Star Quality
Development Phase

In this first month you are going to be feeling yourself out, gauging your fitness level, and formulating your foundation. But first, here are some important tips before you get started.

Never Stretch a Cold Muscle

I constantly see so-called exercise fanatics putting on their running shoes and immediately bending their bodies forward to stretch their hamstrings. Then they proceed to stretch their quads and calves with such self-assured pride that you would think they knew what they were doing. They obviously don't. You never want to stretch a cold muscle.

Before you bend over, twist, reach back, or do anything else that pulls on your muscles and tendons, you've got to warm up and get the blood flowing. Stretching a cold muscle is like stretching cold taffy. Yes, taffy is meant to be malleable. You can bend it, twist it, and flip it around . . . but only when it's slightly warm, making it soft and pliable. If you try to bend a cold piece of taffy in half, it will break. Don't risk an uncomfortable pull, tear, or all-out rip to your muscles or tendons. Warm up, then stretch out!

Warm Up

Before any workout you have to warm up. The warmup gets your blood pumping through your veins and into your muscles. It makes the more intense movements of your workout more effective. It makes your tendons more flexible, minimizing your chances of injury. As you become more aware of your breath, you will feel each deep inhale increasing the oxygen flow throughout your body, giving your muscles energy. The surge of oxygen also fills your brain, giving your body more precise control over its movements. With your entire system moving at a slightly faster pace, your temperature will begin to rise, warming up the body, making it more pliable and prepared for a strenuous workout. The extra heat also helps your body to more effectively burn stored sugars in the creation of energy, allowing for a greater, more consistent calorie burn. Because you are easing your body into exercise as opposed to shocking it into a full-speed run, you will be able to work out longer before getting exhausted. Warming up also minimizes the amount of lactic acid that is unleashed throughout your body, so your muscles won't be as sore the next day.

Once you're all warmed up (which takes about five minutes), it's time to get that body moving!

Postexercise: Stretch It All Out

Why do you feel the need to jump into a fifteen-minute steam shower immediately after a workout, but can't take five minutes to stretch? Believe me, if you don't spend time stretching today, you will be in even more pain tomorrow. You have to get the lactic acid

Model Gazing

True or false: Staring at images of models will help improve your own body image. Well, true if you make sure those models are healthy. Looking at gaunt catwalkers doesn't do anything good for your self-esteem. Tear out a photo of your favorite healthy model and tape it to your fridge for inspiration.

buildup out of your muscles so it doesn't accumulate in one spot and give you some serious cramping tomorrow, the next day, and maybe even the day after that! Stretching won't make the pain completely disappear, but I promise you will be a lot better off if you do it.

Not only does it disperse lactic acid buildup, but stretching also improves your range of motion, making everyday movements—like reaching for a mug on a high shelf or picking up a ball from the ground and throwing it across the yard—that much easier. Stretching makes you more flexible and limber, which can also improve your posture and make you look both thinner and taller. So take a couple of minutes and do the easy stretching exercises.

Month 1

Your workout days this month will be Monday, Tuesday, Thursday, Friday, and Saturday. Take Wednesday and Sunday off. It is a good idea to have one day of rest (you will do only cardio on rest days) in between your resistance workouts in order to give your muscles time to rejuvenate.

Week 1

You will do twenty minutes of aerobic exercise each workout day. This first week the aerobic workout will be walking.

On three of your workout days, you will add resistance training. You will choose from your accessorizing options: four different upper-body moves and four different lower-body moves from chapter 8. Try not to choose the same exercises each day or you will risk overworking and injuring that particular muscle. Instead, select several different exercises each day, targeting different areas. The goal is to work complementary muscles—your triceps and biceps, your quadriceps and hamstrings. Balance is the key to avoiding injury.

In this part of the program you will have to assess your own strength. By trying several of the resistance exercises, you will be able to gauge which of your muscle groups are stronger than others and which are weaker. Because we all have muscles that are more developed than others, some of the exercises will be much easier for you than others may be. Try to balance each workout with both easier and more difficult exercises. Remember, by the end of the month you will have tried them all—lots of times. So you won't be able to avoid any particular exercise just because it is hard or you don't like it for some reason. Besides, why would you want to train unevenly, bulking out some muscles and not others? Train evenly and trust your body. Don't push yourself too far, but push yourself just far enough so that you experience the effects of the workout and your body evolves.

Week 2

You will do twenty minutes of aerobic exercise each workout day. Continue to walk, but add hills—or change it up and start biking.

On three days, you will also do resistance work—five upper-body and five lower-body exercises from the list.

Pounding the pavement is more exhausting than pounding the belt of your treadmill. The average exerciser tends to let herself off a little easier on a treadmill, walking slightly slower while absorbed in watching reruns or talk shows or listening to music. But more than simply preventing you from letting yourself slack off on the treadmill, exercising outside has been proven to be more physically challenging.

First of all, you don't have the motorized belt to push your body forward. While outside, as you attempt, without mechanical

Learn How to Read Your Body's Needs

It's easy for the advanced exerciser to take it up a notch or for the beginner to ease off a bit by adding or subtracting reps or speeding up or slowing down your pace. Just be honest with yourself and listen to your body's signals. If, at the end of your sets, your muscle still doesn't feel fatigued, you are strong enough to take that exercise up a notch. If, on the other hand, you feel pangs of pain or muscle pulls, or you are simply unable to get through a set, you need to ease off a bit. When you push yourself too much, one way that your body copes is by calling to other stronger muscles to contribute. If you start to look to other areas of your body to do the exercise, that is a warning that you are near your end. Some common muscles that come into play are the back, the thighs, even the neck. You might also notice that you want to swing or bounce into a move. Those are ways of tempting injury. If you want your body to efficiently change through fitness, be mindful of its movements.

assistance, to propel yourself forward—one foot in front of the other—you have wind resistance pushing you back. And don't forget that most terrain isn't 100 percent flat; there is usually some sort of an up- or downgrade forcing your muscles to work in a slightly different, constantly changing motion.

It's said that you have to set your treadmill to at least a 1 percent grade in order to emulate the angle that you might get while walking on the street. But again, when outside do you consistently walk at a steady and barely noticeable 1 percent grade? Probably not. Outside, the ground is uneven; there are hills (however slight) to climb and descend, curbs to jump, and cracks to hurdle. Your natural environment outside offers a much more intense, varied, and interesting routine that always keeps you on your toes. So take it outside!

Work Out with Music

Studies show that exercising with music can actually make you want to move faster and push yourself harder than you would if you were exercising in silence.

Week 3

You will do thirty minutes of aerobic exercise each workout day—walking/jogging in five-minute increments: four minutes of walking/one minute of jogging, repeated six times. On three days, you will also do resistance work—six different upper-body moves and six different lower-body moves.

On-the-Go Exercise

One-Legged Plank

This exercise works your butt, waist, chest, shoulders, thighs—basically it's full-body sculpting in one move.

- Start in plank position (that is, the top of the push-up, with your entire body weight supported by your hands and toes). Keep your body straight, making sure that your butt isn't sticking up or sagging. Keep your hands shoulder-width apart.

- Keep your arms and legs straight and lift one leg a few inches off the ground (go as high as you can without engaging the lower back).

- Bend your elbows and lower your body to the bottom of a push-up (without releasing your chest to the ground).

- Press your arms straight, but keep your leg up.

- Bend the knee of your elevated leg into your chest, toward your stomach.

- Straighten your leg and keep it elevated off the ground.

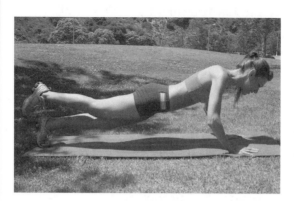

- Push your elevated leg up a few inches, starting the movement in your butt and pushing through to your heel.

- Repeat 10 times.

- Switch legs and repeat.

Log On and Lose Weight

If your food and exercise journal isn't motivating you enough to move, think about going online and starting a blog. There is something to say for speaking candidly about your struggle and knowing that someone out there is listening. You get to voice your plight while becoming a source of inspiration for others. Readers of your blog will start to log on regularly to gauge your success. They will cheerlead for you and track your waistline, too. Cutting calories, sticking with your exercise program, and staying positive become easier when you are answering to more than just yourself—countless people across the country and around the world will be checking in on you.

More than faceless groupies following your daily ups and downs, you will find an instant support system of other bloggers—people like you who are also struggling with unsupportive family members, frustrating plateaus, ex-boyfriend-inspired gorging, and all of the other trials and tribulations that you are physically and mentally experiencing.

Going online can allow you to be as anonymous or as known as you like. You can publish photos, be honest about your weight, elaborate on your short-term and long-term goals. You will also learn that you can track yourself. What prompted you to eat that bag of cookies? What time of day did you feel energized during your exercise? Are you really working as hard as you think you are?

Need another reason to take it outside? You'll avoid boredom. Cycling is pretty much boredom proof. It gets you out of the steamy Spinning room and allows you to *really* ride through forests and along the beach, to climb up hills and race down—imagery was never my thing. You get to breathe fresh air instead of recycled sweat-soaked air. Spinning your wheels outside also burns more than 800 calories an hour while sculpting your butt and thighs without impacting the knees.

Week 4

You will do thirty minutes of aerobic exercise each workout day—walking/jogging in five-minute increments: three minutes of walking/two minutes of jogging, repeated six times.

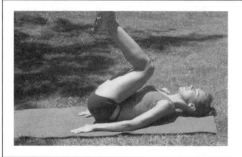

On three days, you will also do resistance work—seven different upper-body moves and seven different lower-body moves.

Real Woman, Real Story

Lisa Vidal was thirty-six when we started working together. She was already thin and in pretty good shape, but she wanted to get more definition and muscle tone. She wanted to get strong. She needed to increase her energy and stop feeling so tired all the time. She used to work out with a trainer at the gym. The problem for her was that there was a lot of socializing going on and too many breaks. That's basically the atmosphere at every gym. Before you know it, your hour is up and you don't feel you got a workout. You barely even squeezed out a drop of sweat.

We immediately jumped into a routine of biking and running—a lot. To change up her cardio routine and for almost instant results, we skipped. It's is a great workout! We would do quick side skips through the neighborhood to work her legs and that spot where the butt and leg meet. We also did

Rolling Crunch

This exercise works your entire core.

- Lie on your back with your knees bent, feet on the ground.
- Bring your knees into your chest so that your shins are parallel to the ground.
- Rest your hands behind your head for support.
- Lift your head and chest to a sit-up position.
- Roll your butt slightly up off the ground so that you are balancing on your back.
- Touch your knees to your elbows.
- Keeping your elbows and knees connected, slowly rock back and forth.
- Do 20 reps (one rep is a full back-and-forth motion).

high-rep weight training using mat exercises and free weights, but focused on traditional exercises like lunges, sit-ups, and push-ups. We used tables and chairs as supports. The concept may seem simple, but what it taught Lisa is that you can exercise anywhere. You don't need a gym membership or fancy equipment to get an intense, full-body workout. You can work out alone. You can work out at home. You can work out with friends. You can work out while traveling. No equipment needed.

For Lisa we built a fitness foundation, then we prepared her body for pregnancy—her third. After she gave birth, her workouts remained basically the same.

Now, with three kids, it's hard for Lisa to get in her program on a regular basis, so when she can't do her traditional workout, she incorporates exercise wherever and whenever she can. Her kids are into soccer, so she might run around on the field with them, then drop down for a set of sit-ups and push-ups. She rides her bike and swims—anything to keep cardio interesting since she doesn't like that part of working out. We may not work out together like we used to, but she tells me that my voice remains in her head, pushing her up that hill on her bike, counting out her sit-ups.

You need to find what motivates you. You may not like cardio, or you may hate lunges or crunches, so find a way to make it fun. At the end of every workout, you will be reminded that it's worth it.

Dump Your Fat Pants

Get rid of old clothes that don't fit anymore. Why keep fat pants around? You aren't going back! Besides, you need room for your new wardrobe.

Star Quality
Production Phase

It's time to start getting more specific. In this second month you will continue with your basic routine, but you will also begin to hone in on your body-type goals by accessorizing with a little glitz and glam. We will add more cardio and resistance to keep changing it up and challenging your body.

To increase the Star Quality body burn, we will also speed things up a bit. Moving faster through your workout will build your endurance, work off more calories and, obviously, shorten your workout time.

A study in the *Journal of Applied Physiology* showed that when cyclists did six sprint intervals (thirty seconds all out followed by four minutes at a slower pace) instead of half an hour of straight riding, they doubled their endurance and could travel twice the distance before becoming exhausted. As with cycling, when it comes to walking or running, pace matters. According to a study from the University of Alberta, Edmonton, those who walk at a moderately intense measured speed enjoyed more than double the cardio fitness and blood pressure improvement than those who walked at their own pace for ten thousand steps.

You can incorporate interval training into your walking routine to keep your heart rate elevated and calories burning off. For example, once you are warmed up, you might run all out for two minutes, then drop it down a shade with an active recovery by speed walking for two minutes. Then repeat, repeat, repeat.

Circuit training allows you to squeeze in more exercise in less time by upping the intensity, so you immediately move from one muscle group to the next without recovery time. With circuit training you might run for five minutes, focus on abs for five minutes, do lunges for five minutes, then do push-ups and seated dips to hone in on your arms for five minutes—then repeat the process in a constantly moving circuit.

Another way to get the most out of your workout is to break it up. Researchers at the University of Missouri–Columbia discovered that taking a quick breather during a training session minimizes triglyceride levels (translation: fat) in the bloodstream. The level of the most effective fat-clearing enzyme found in the blood increases the most during the postworkout recovery phase. The study shows that the more frequently you rest, the more chance you have for your body to release the enzyme into your bloodstream. But don't go overboard. You should work out continuously for thirty minutes before taking a twenty-minute break—which is when you can do your resistance training. Or, if you are out on a bike ride, stop for a picnic or get off your bike and walk around to take in the scenery.

Taking it outside heightens the benefits of your fitness program and makes it even more enjoyable. Getting fresh air may also encourage you to be more active. Studies show that people who regularly hit the trails for hikes and other outdoor activities are twice as likely to do thirty minutes of exercise most days than those who stick to exercising indoors.

Accidental Exercise

Sit Up Straight

Sit up straight to help strengthen your core. Sitting up forces all the supporting muscles in your stomach to stack up and engage each fiber—making them stronger, tighter, and naturally flexed.

Get Psyched

Grab a Friend

Work out with a friend and you will be seven times less likely to ditch your routine.

Month 2

Your workout days this month will be Monday, Tuesday, Thursday, Friday, and Saturday. Take Wednesday and Sunday off. Four of these days will include resistance work.

Week 1

You will do thirty-five minutes of aerobic exercise each workout day—walking/jogging in five-minute increments: two minutes of walking/three minutes of jogging, repeated seven times. On Monday, Tuesday, Thursday, and Saturday, you will also do resistance work—eight different upper-body moves and eight different lower-body moves.

Up the Ante

Time Your Meals

Research suggests that waiting to eat until after your workout can motivate your body to tap into your fat stores and burn more calories while exercising. On the other hand, if you are feeling famished, eat! Hunger to the point of weakness will slow you down and make you burn less calories.

Got Fifteen Minutes?

You can get an intense calorie-burning workout in no time at all.

Intervals are an excellent way to take advantage of every second you've got to sizzle away excess calories. Don't be one of those people who say, "I have only fifteen minutes. Oh well, I guess I have to skip my exercise today." No! Even fifteen minutes can make a dent. And when you are trying to drop fat and tone muscle, those fifteen minutes will be well worth the sweat and shower. Maximize your fifteen minutes by following this simple fast fitness plan:

0–3 minutes:	Warm up with a fast walk
3–6 minutes:	Jog
6–7 minutes:	Slow down to a fast walk
7–10 minutes:	Run
10–11 minutes:	Slow down to a fast walk
11–13 minutes:	Run up a hill or up stairs, or just run all out
13–14 minutes:	Slow down to a fast walk
14–15 minutes:	Cool down with a slow walk

Week 2

You will do thirty-five minutes of aerobic exercise each workout day—walking/jogging in five-minute increments: two minutes of walking/three minutes of jogging, repeated seven times.

On Monday, Tuesday, Thursday, and Saturday, you will also do resistance work—nine different upper-body moves and nine different lower-body moves.

On-the-Go Exercise
Tabletop Pull-Through

This exercise works your shoulders, arms, abs, butt, and legs.

- Sit up straight on a mat with your knees bent, feet flat on the ground hip-width apart, toes pointing forward.
- Place your hands flat on the ground approximately 12 inches behind your butt, fingers facing forward.
- Press your weight into your hands and feet as you lift your butt and hips up into the air in the shape of a tabletop. Your face should be pointing forward and slightly up.
- Bend your legs and lower your butt down to an inch above the ground. Keep your butt off the ground. Your hands should remain flat on the ground. Though your toes will raise up, your heels should remain firmly planted.

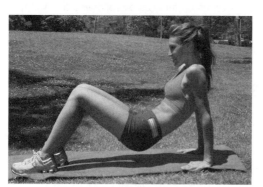

- Hold in that position with your arms straight and your legs bent for four seconds.
- Return to the tabletop position and hold for another four seconds.
- Repeat 15 times.

Week 3

You will do forty minutes of aerobic exercise each workout day—walking/jogging in five-minute increments: two minutes of walking/three minutes of jogging, repeated eight times.

On Monday, Tuesday, Thursday, and Saturday, you will also do resistance work—ten different upper-body moves and ten different lower-body moves.

Week 4

You will do forty minutes of aerobic exercise each workout day—walking/ jogging in five-minute increments: two minutes of walking/three minutes of jogging, repeated eight times.

On Monday, Tuesday, Thursday, and Saturday, you will also do resistance work—eleven different upper-body moves and eleven different lower-body moves.

Accidental Exercise

Exercise at Work

Some jobs leave you sedentary all day long. Others allow for constant activity. Does your career lead to office butt or trim thighs? According to the American Council on Exercise, some jobs force you to get up on your feet and move it.

- Mail carriers take an average of 18,904 steps each day
- Custodians take 12,991 steps
- Restaurant servers take 10,087 steps
- Nurses take 8,648 steps
- Lawyers take 5,062 steps
- Teachers take 4,726 steps
- Wear a pedometer to work tomorrow and see how your job measures up.

Real Woman, Real Story

Kathy Poncher, a fifty-eight-year-old designer, wanted to get in better shape. She had worked out with different trainers all her life, but the strain that was placed on her weak back (she was already missing a couple of discs) would cause it to be blown out within the first few weeks. Instead of tempting more pain and injury, she ran forty miles a week through the mountains on her own (the only form of exercise that she found didn't put stress on her back). While running was keeping her slim, Kathy wanted to build strength.

To change up her regular routine without aggravating her back, I placed her in specific poses that we would then build on. I would have Kathy kneel down in a certain position that would target a muscle building area without causing any tension to other areas. Without the muscle pain, her running increased from forty miles to fifty-five miles per week as she began to train for a half marathon! But we still needed to change her cardio program in order to keep it interesting and keep her focused.

Bike riding seemed to me to be the perfect workout for Kathy. But Kathy had no interest in falling, and, due to her back injury, she was worried about riding a bike. We worked on riding properly—on balance and stride. She learned when to pedal and when not to in order to avoid injury and make the most out of her workout. What she realized is that when you are coasting, your feet should be at the same level—not one up and one down. The position in which you sit is also important. It's best to sit at the front of the seat when you are going uphill and farther back when you are going downhill to balance out the bike. In addition to improving her basic technique, we balanced out Kathy's body by adding strength and muscle to her calves. Knowing how to exercise, creating balance in both the body and the exercise program, and understanding the

Demi Moore and Motivation

Working out with friends can help keep you motivated. Demi Moore surrounds herself with friends, even when she's staying at her home in Idaho. There is always a revolving door of famous faces, including John Travolta and Kelly Preston, Goldie Hawn and Kurt Russell, Sylvester Stallone, Cindy Crawford, and Meg Ryan. One snowy afternoon it was time to hit the "gym"—the great white outdoors. Demi's celebrity friends thought we were crazy, but we convinced them to gear up in snowshoes and get outside. We all had a great workout and smiled and laughed the entire time. Yes, it was exercise, but it felt more like play. Sometimes, working out with a group of friends forces you to dig down deeper and push yourself further than you normally would have. Another example: Once Demi and I accidentally got caught in a snowstorm while on a run six miles from her home. That time it was the stinging pain and the snow whipping against our faces that motivated us to run faster.

basic positions and body alignment makes it more fun and minimizes the risk of injury. Proper technique and body balance enabled Kathy to work out consistently without injury—rather than exercise for three months, get injured, and take off a year, during which she experienced daily pain. Once Kathy was ready to really work out using a bike, we would ride for an hour at a time at different speeds and inclines, in different terrains and places. It was an intense workout, but it was also a blast.

But you can't get a complete workout just from riding a bike, so when we rode through the mountains we would often stop and do push-ups. We avoided lunges because they can create too much back tension, but we easily worked around it. We would use trees for support or we would use towels to create resistance. Branches worked, too. Rarely did we use traditional weights, since we were able to get all the resistance we needed from Kathy's own body or the things we had around us while in the mountains during our bike rides.

When off the bike and trekking along a trail, we'd mix it up by running up and down stairs and hills, and we also changed speeds from a slow jog to an all-out sprint. Kathy quickly realized that she didn't need a gym, that she had a circuit within her body and in her environment.

Kathy is great at pushing herself, so that I don't have to encourage her too much. We both know her limitations, which has allowed for great bodily change without ever causing an injury.

Of course, as is the case for so many other regular exercisers, when her alarm goes off in the morning, often Kathy's first thought is to roll over and go back to sleep. But she doesn't. Getting outside helps. She slips on her shoes and moves her body in the crisp air. Pretty soon she is far away from home and she may as well keep it up instead of turning back and giving up. When you are outside you have things to see, scents to smell, fresh air to breathe.

Kathy prefers to run without an MP3 player plugged into her ears. Sometimes she recites poetry, making it up as she goes, her issues spewing out. Exercise is a creative outlet for Kathy. Since writing down her poems while running through the hills is not an option, she bought a tiny voice recorder that she takes with her to record her thoughts, songs, and poems. When she runs for long distances, the chatter in her mind quiets and her consciousness comes out and is fully present. Getting to that place of calm can take anywhere from twenty to forty minutes. At first it can be a real struggle to mentally get going. Sometimes she just forces herself along as she reviews the day.

Running is emotionally freeing for Kathy. She gets outside and burns off the emotional stuff as well as the extra calories.

I once asked Kathy why she exercises. Her response was "Why do we breathe?" She works out because it feels so good after. Exercise also happens to be the only thing that has ever worked for her hot flashes. It keeps them in check and keeps her going. For Kathy, the purpose of exercise is more than having a great body. It is more of an internal cleansing of the body and mind that nourishes and refreshes the spirit. She feels that it is all about trying to have more clarity and get in tune with herself.

On-the-Go Exercise

Got Ten Minutes?

Working out for ten minutes is worth your while. Three ten-minute cardio sessions can give you the same health benefits as one thirty-minute session.

11

Star Quality Postproduction Phase

Your body is now getting used to the program, so it's time to up the ante. I know, you have gotten comfortable, but if you want to continue making significant change in your body, you have to increase the intensity, raise your heart rate, and challenge your muscles.

This month we will focus on compound movements that work multiple areas of your body at once, in order to be as efficient as possible, as well as isolations, so we can hone in on particular body parts.

A recent study confirmed that regular aerobic exercise (loosely defined as three hours a week) increases brain volume in older adults, which translates to better concentration and memory. In younger people this can help stave off mental decline, which starts in your twenties.

Want a surefire way to stick to your routine? Have fun with it! Keeping it interesting and something that you look forward to every day will make you miss it if you miss it.

The way the resistance exercises are going to be handled this final month is as follows:

Monday, Wednesday, and Friday

Compound movements: Quadriceps and hamstrings—pliés, presses, step-ups, jump squats, lunges

Isolation: Chest, shoulders, and triceps—presses Abs—full crunches

Tuesday and Thursday

Compound movements: Inner and outer thighs and glutes—plié squats, skiing squats, lunges

Isolation: Biceps—curls Abs—working the obliques (the stomach muscles that wrap around your sides)

Every other week you will flip-flop your program so that your Monday, Wednesday, and Friday exercises are done on Tuesday and Thursday, and vice versa.

Don't give up now, or you will risk losing everything that you have worked for! Believe me, I have seen it, even with celebs.

Month 3

Your workout days this month will be Monday, Tuesday, Wednesday, Thursday, Friday, and Saturday; take Sunday off. You will do resistance work on five of these days.

Week 1

You will do forty-five minutes of aerobic exercise each workout day—walking/jogging in five-minute increments: 1 minute of walking/four minutes of jogging, repeated nine times.

On Monday, Tuesday, Wednesday, Friday, and Saturday, you will also do resistance work—twelve different upper-body moves and twelve different lower-body moves.

Get Psyched

Crunch

If you start daydreaming about sweets, distract yourself by doing something physical—like crunches in front of the TV. The endorphins released and the calories burned will actually banish your cravings.

Week 2

You will do forty-five minutes of aerobic exercise each workout day—walking/jogging in five-minute increments: one minute of walking/four minutes of jogging, repeated nine times.

On Monday, Tuesday, Wednesday, Friday, and Saturday, you will also do resistance work—thirteen different upper-body moves and thirteen different lower-body moves.

Pace Matters

Remember that pace matters. Some people wrongly believe that as long as you are going the same distance and clocking the same mileage running and walking, will burn the same amount of calories. Wrong! Running gets your heart pumping, your blood flowing, and your muscles firing at a much greater intensity than walking. When you run, you are leaping off the ground with each step, while the motion of walking is just pushing the feet forward, one in front of the other. The fact is that for every mile you walk, you would have burned through about twice the calories had you run it.

Outside Awareness

Exercising outside offers great sun exposure. But you do need to be careful not to soak up too many potentially harmful rays. Be sure to wear sunscreen when working out outside. Even during winter months and cool days, protect yourself. High altitudes and UVB rays penetrating thin clouds can unknowingly do some serious damage. Studies show that spray-on sunscreens are better than creams because you are less likely to miss a spot or unevenly spread it into wrinkles and creases. And don't forget about the your hands, calves, neck, and ears. Baseball caps also are great for extra coverage for the face.

Don't use the sun as an excuse to stay in or avoid exercise altogether. If you are really concerned, work out in the morning before the sun beats down, or in the evening as the sun is beginning to fade away.

Up the Ante

Do Your Upper- and Lower-Body Exercises at the Same Time

Once you have gained enough strength and balance to add a little extra to your resistance-training routine, try this challenge—combine your upper- and lower-body exercises into one calorie-singeing, heart-pounding, stability-challenging exercise. Doing a lunge (which works the legs) while doing a bicep curl, or doing a wall sit and a shoulder press, makes more muscles work at the same time. As a result, your balance is tested (which also works more muscles—those stabilizing muscles), you up your calorie burn, and you increase your heart rate. Not to mention that you save time.

Week 3

You will do fifty minutes of aerobic exercise each workout day—walking/jogging in five-minute increments: one minute of walking/four minutes of jogging, repeated ten times.

On Monday, Tuesday, Wednesday, Friday, and Saturday, you will also do resistance work—fourteen different upper-body moves and fourteen different lower-body moves.

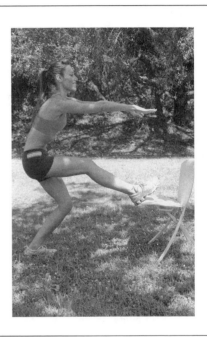

On-the-Go Exercise

One-Legged Squat

This exercise works your legs, butt, and core.

- Stand facing a chair or a bench about 2 feet away. Place one foot on the chair and keep your standing leg straight.

- Extend your arms straight out as if you are reaching for something.

- Slowly bend your standing leg, sticking out your butt but keeping your chest lifted, as if you are about to sit down.

- Be careful not to let the knee of your standing leg bend past the front of your toes.

- Repeat 10–15 times for one set. Then switch legs and repeat.

Week 4

You will do fifty minutes of aerobic exercise each workout day—walking/jogging in five-minute increments: one minute of walking/four minutes of jogging, repeated ten times.

On Monday, Tuesday, Wednesday, Friday, and Saturday, you will also do resistance work—fifteen different upper-body moves and fifteen different lower-body moves.

Feeling the Calorie Burn?
Maybe Not . . .

How many calories do you think are you burning during your one-hour cardio workout? Well, now you can find out.

Belly dancing: 290 calories

Bike riding on the street (or anywhere but a trail): 640 calories

Circuit training (high intensity, combining cardio and resistance): 510 calories

Cross-country skiing: 510 calories

Doing tai chi: 255 calories

Gardening: 290 calories

Golfing (carrying your clubs and walking instead of taking the cart): 290 calories

Hiking: 385 calories

Jumping rope: 640 calories

Kayaking: 320 calories

Mountain biking: 545 calories

Playing basketball: 290 calories

Playing soccer: 640 calories

Running: 640 calories

Running stairs: 960 calories

Swimming laps: 450 calories

Trail running: 575 calories

Walking at a fast pace: 320 calories

Walking at a moderate pace: 245 calories

Take-It-Outside Philosophy

Remember that even a casual stroll can turn into a workout. Try to walk at a quick pace. Once you are sure your muscles are warmed up, stop every few minutes and do ten lunges or reverse lunges on each leg. If you come across a bench, do step-ups, seated dips, or angled push-ups off the edge. A steep driveway or a set of stairs provides the perfect opportunity to run up and down a couple of times. Repeat strength exercises three times during your walk to get the most out of them and really work your muscles.

Your environment is the best gym there is. You have an interval course laid out for you. All you have to do is view your surroundings

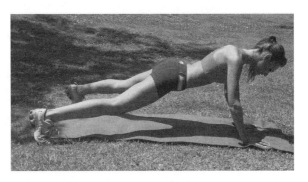

Naomi Watts's Motivation to Get through the Tough Times— Joking and Competition

Sometimes Naomi's workouts became mentally tough. To deal with this, she had her brother or friends work out with us. This technique worked well for her because of her competitive nature. Naomi and her brother would challenge and joke with each other throughout the workout.

slightly differently. Look at the grass as a soft pad for sit-ups. Trees and solid fences offer a stable foundation to lean against for wall sits. Bleachers are perfect for step-ups. Benches couldn't be better for seated dips and push-ups. Sidewalks and trails are great places to do lunges and squats, not to mention your cardio—running, biking, even skipping and jumping.

More than a great place for exercising, the outdoors is calming, even during intense physical activity. Studies show that just being around green trees and grass can chemically calm the brain. What else can I say? Take it outside!

Real Woman, Real Story

Marla is a comedian. She performs live and on a television show called *Girls Behaving Badly*. We were matched up by *Allure* magazine, which was doing an article about six-week body makeovers. I was the trainer. She was the woman who wanted to lose twenty-five pounds. What was interesting about Marla was that she had always been athletic and she was pretty sure she knew a lot about how to exercise properly. In fact, she worked out regularly, walking three to four miles a day plus going to the gym. But she was also a sugar addict and found comfort in food.

Marla grew up in a household where food was treated as a Band-Aid for pain, anger, and sadness. As she so comedically put it, "If I fell off my bicycle, my grandma would defrost a brisket." Her perception of food was always "What better way to get over anger than pizza and cookies?" She would tell me about the "emergency cake" that her mom kept for Marla to nibble on as a kid.

When the *Allure* article presented itself, Marla had just moved from New York to Los Angeles; she didn't want to use the chubby excuse for missing out on good acting parts and comedy gigs. The

Don't Sabotage Yourself

As you may or may not be experiencing around this time, exercisers are more likely to fall into a rut and relapse into old unhealthy ways as soon as they see improvement in their body and lifestyle. You finally fit into your skinny jeans or you are constantly being complimented on how great you look, and you think, Well, this must have worked; now I can go back to my old ways. I can indulge in my favorite things again! I have succeeded. If this is you, believe me when I tell you that very soon you will no longer be able to pour yourself into your skinny jeans, and you will be forced to put on your fat pants again.

If you want to reward yourself for your success, have one little indulgent something—a glass of champagne, a cookie, an extra day off from your exercise program. But please, do not go back to your old ways. You will have wasted your time. Let's keep the positive momentum going strong! You have done so well. That flab that used to bulge over your bra strap is gone—or at least it's on its way out! That loose fatty skin that used to flap around on the underside of your upper arms is now tight and toned. You look amazing! Keep it up.

first thing I told her was to get rid of the cheese. She was eating way too much of it. I asked her to write down what she ate, and she admittedly cheated . . . for a while. But soon she decided to take advantage of this opportunity and focus. She had to be honest with herself and with me.

I put her on a program, taught her about heart rate, and helped her to lose the "muffin top" that hung over the waistband of her pants.

Marla likes to tell people that I intimidated her at first. She was this typical New Yorker with a tough personality, always cracking a joke to avoid difficult issues. I didn't laugh—though it was sometimes hard not to—because it was time to get serious in order to get in shape.

We added an incline or a jog to her daily walk. Sometimes she hiked. She also incorporated resistance work. At first she was against resistance training, believing that lifting weight would bulk her up. But as soon as she started noticing results, she became a believer.

I reminded her that what's important isn't the size; it's how your clothes fit. Freed from the numbers, Marla went down a size and bought her first pair of "fancy jeans." She got rid of her fat pants and looked forward, not back.

After the six weeks that we trained together, Marla went back on the road, but she sticks with her program and continues to maintain her exercise routine. Workouts are built into her day—they have to be, or she wouldn't get to them.

Being on tour can be hard for Marla. Traveling in general is rough on a diet. In Marla's case, she would have a cocktail and it would trigger her to go back to her old food ways. She decided to stop using food to medicate. Instead she wanted to feel her emotions, feel the anxiety. Now if she feels like snacking she will have an apple with peanut butter, a frozen yogurt with fresh fruit, or a protein bar—a small one. Marla has embraced portion control and realized that she doesn't need so much food.

Working out has made Marla feel better about herself. She no longer sees herself as funny and fat. Marla has empowered herself. Now, when she looks out at an audience, she likes how men respond to a funny, loud woman who they also think is hot. Amazing what exercising can do for you.

12

Star Quality Maintenance

You did it. I'm proud of you. Getting in shape is a huge accomplishment! But you aren't done yet. As I said before, fitness is a lifestyle. Don't give up now. You have worked so hard, dragged yourself out of bed, eliminated who knows how many toxins from your body, broken down and melted away inches of fat, built up muscle, and basked in the glory of health. If you give up now, all that hard work will be for naught. You will balloon again, returning to the place you started, if not going even further into the dumps and getting fatter. Not really what you had in mind, is it?

This maintenance program isn't as intense as the three-month, get-your-butt-in-gear, boot camp–style program you just completed, so you can let out a nice big sigh of relief.

Your program, from now on, consists of (1) five days of aerobic training, (2) three days of strength conditioning, and (3) stretching.

If you have a big event and need to slip into a slinky number, go back to the third-month program and work off a few straggling inches or pounds. Just don't let yourself fall into a rut. When you're not feeling immediate pressure to trim down and tone up, follow the second-month program. Continue to accessorize with your cardio and strength options to change it up and add variety. Variety

---

Got Ten Minutes?

Burn fat and calories with a quick stair workout. It is a great way to trim and tone the butt and thighs while getting your heart going. Here's how:

Minute 0–1: Casually walk up and down a flight (or several flights) of stairs. Be sure to swing your arms as you would if you were running, keeping your back tall, your chin and eyes forward and slightly up, and your tailbone slightly tucked.

Minutes 1–3: Starting with your left foot, step up and back down (without turning around) on the first step. Repeat this ten times. Then, starting with the left foot, step up and back down on the second step. Repeat this ten times. Continue going up the steps for two minutes.

Minutes 3–5: You are going to do a "box step" on the bottom step. Step your right foot up on the step. Then raise your body up and cross your left foot over your right foot, placing it down on the right side of your right foot. Now pick up your right foot and place it on the ground. Pick up your left foot and return it to the left side of the right foot—in normal standing stance—on the ground. Repeat as quickly as you can for two minutes.

Minutes 5–7: Repeat the box step on the opposite side, leading with the left foot.

Minutes 7–8: Step up onto the bottom step with your right foot. As your shift your weight up onto your right foot, shoot your left knee up so that your left foot is at the level between your waist and your knee of your right straight leg. Keep your right foot planted on the step and release your left foot back down to the ground. Repeat on the same side.

Minutes 8–9: Repeat the step-up on the opposite side, with the left foot planted up on the step.

Minutes 9–10: Run up the stairs as fast as you can without tripping. Quickly walk down the stairs. Repeat for one minute.

Cool down by walking for two minutes.

---

will help you improve your fitness level and eliminate exercise boredom.

You should now have a good understanding of the exercises, so trust yourself to mix and match the elements of your program depending on your goal. Keep it up. You're doing a great job.

Star Quality Sport-Specific Fitness

Are you training for a triathlon? Do you want to improve your yoga asanas? Are your surfing skills in need of a tune-up? Could your basketball game use a boost? There are exercises you can do to target the specific muscle groups that help increase your ability, agility, endurance, range of motion, oxygen intake, and stamina to perform better at your favorite fitness activity.

In this section I will give you exercises and tips on how to improve your game, whatever game that is. The focus will be on functional exercises that train your movements, as opposed to training your muscles. To really be a pro you need to be able to catch, push off, toss, weave, and duck—without thinking about how to do the movement. Training your movements gets your body accustomed to positioning and manipulating your body in a specific way. It is not so much about making a muscle strong but rather about making a movement strong.

Skiing

You may not be able to ski year-round, but you can train your muscles to perform at their peak skiing level even during the off-season. Supplementing these exercises with your skiing during the ski season will focus your training, fine-tuning your muscles and preparing them for race days.

Functional training will target specific muscle groups by mimicking the movements of your sport. I don't care how much weight you can press or how many lunges you can do if you don't have the movement endurance to support a high-speed race.

With skiing we will focus our attention on two things: balance and strength. Spending time learning how to stay stable will help you move more accurately, take sharper turns, hold off-center positions longer. Arguably more important, stability work will minimize your chances of taking a bad fall and injuring yourself, potentially taking you out of the game. Working on strength will help support the muscles that are holding your body in balance, while increasing your ability to place a large amount of force on your downhill leg for extended periods of time.

Do your regular daily foundation routine of cardio and resistance work, then tack on these extra exercises, adding four extra movements to your resistance training. If it's too much for you, replace four resistance moves with these ski-specific alternatives. These exercises are done the same way for all body types.

Downhill Lunge

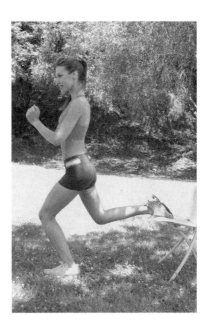

The downhill lunge mimics the movement of your legs when navigating moguls, including the pressure on your quadriceps and knees. It gives you that same muscle burn and total leg strain.

POSITION
- Pretend you're wearing ski boots.
- Stand with the backs of your legs approximately 24 inches away from a chair, a step, or a bench.
- Stand on one leg.

MOVEMENT
- Bend your other leg and place the top of that foot on the step behind you.
- Slowly and with control, bend your standing leg to a 90-degree angle. As you bend down, the leg that is elevated on the step will also lower at the knee.
- Do 3 sets of 12 reps on each leg, for a total of 6 sets.

Up the Ante

Add Weight

Hold a 5-pound dumbbell in your hands. Keep the weight centered against your stomach as you do the movement.

Ski Squat

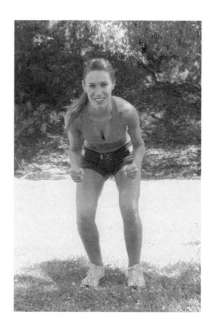

Though you may be going down a steep hill with gravity supporting your downward movement, you still have to maintain control and often negotiate sharp turns. The ski squat mimics that turning movement as you press your weight down onto the outside ski.

POSITION
- Stand with your feet a few inches apart, your knees slightly bent, and your torso slightly angled forward from your waist.
- Keep both knees slightly bent, shift your center of balance, and slide one foot out to the side (consider this to be your outside skiing leg).

MOVEMENT
- As you extend your leg, bend that leg even farther down, to a 90-degree angle. Plant that foot approximately 3 feet from your standing foot.
- Push your extended foot away from its new spot and return it to the original position with only a slightly bent knee.
- Repeat on the opposite side.
- Remember, you are mimicking the skiing motion. Make sure that you never stand up straight; keep your knees slightly bent and your torso slightly forward, bending from your waist.
- Do 3 sets of 6 reps on each side, for a total of 6 sets.

Hamstring Curl

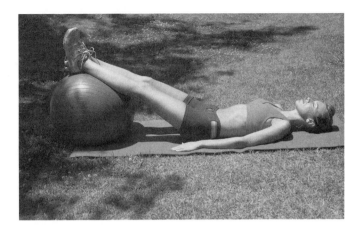

This might not look like something you would do on the slopes, but the movement will strengthen your hamstrings in order to fend off knee problems. By raising your hips off the ground, you will be placing some focus on your core. This exercise also promotes stability since you will be moving on an unstable surface. Be sure not to work your back. Stay focused on your hamstrings, glutes, and abs.

POSITION
- Lie on your back on a mat with your arms at your sides, and your legs extended out and resting on top of a fitness ball.

MOVEMENT
- Lift your hips up so that your legs are almost straight, with your heels digging into the ball.
- Keep your hips up and roll the ball toward your body with your feet until the bottoms of your feet are on top of the ball.
- Without dropping your hips any closer to the ground, roll your feet back out to the straight starting position.
- Do 3 sets of 20 reps.

Leg Recovery

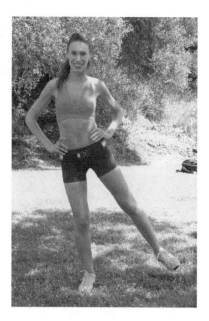

Individual leg stability helps prevent injury and maintain strength. When a skier catches an edge or hits a rock or a stick in the snow, it is easy to lose balance on that foot. Leg recovery exercises help condition skiers to quickly regain stability on the other foot, helping to minimize the risk of a fall.

POSITION
- Stand with your feet shoulder-width apart.
- Slightly bend your knees and angle your body slightly forward from your waist.
- Place your hands on your hips.

MOVEMENT
- Lift your left leg straight up off the ground, extending it out to your side (do not bend your leg).
- Return your left leg to the starting position.
- Repeat until you complete one set (15 to 25 reps).
- Switch legs and repeat.
- Do 3 sets with each leg.

Rowing/Canoeing/Kayaking

If you live near water, chances are you have enjoyed boating. Taking an afternoon to row to a nearby private island to have your own *Gilligan's Island* experience for a few hours is also a popular vacation activity. Regardless of how often you practice the rowing sports, it is important to train the specific muscles utilized in the repetitive movements to improve your paddling ability and minimize your risk of overuse injuries.

If you are not a frequent rower, you will notice soreness in muscles that you may not even have realized existed. So how do you avoid the unwanted muscle awareness? Tone those typically unused muscles. Rowing, canoeing, and kayaking are fundamentally upper-body activities. In prepping the body for the repetitive paddling action, the primary goal is to strengthen the muscles used. The secondary goal is to strengthen the opposing muscle groups in order to balance the body and maintain alignment. Remember, overworking the abs can put undue stress on the opposing muscle group—the back. Overworking the triceps can aggravate the opposing muscle group—the biceps.

The first muscle group we need to be aware of is the back. Proper rowing movement requires that you extend your core and contract your back muscles. As you reach your arms forward to row, you compress your back, placing a lot of stress on those injury-prone muscles. The last thing you want to do is throw out your back midrow miles from shore.

We will focus on two back exercises and one ab exercise (for muscular balance) to prep the back for rowing, canoeing, and kayaking.

Seated Bent-Over Row, Elbows In

Although this is a rowing motion and the movement is in your arms, the focus is on your middle and upper back. As you row, you contract the back, squeezing the muscles together and therefore strengthening them. This exercise both mimics the rowing motion and helps to strengthen your back muscles in a controlled environment without any unexpected variables. For exercise instructions, please see page 137.

Seated Bent-Over Row, Elbows Out

Similar to the seated bent-over row, elbows in, this is a rowing motion, and while the movement is in your arms, the focus is on your mid-back and shoulders. There are so many small but important muscles in your back that help support your larger muscles. Tweaking exercises by changing an angle or making a slight rotation targets a different group of small supportive muscles. As you row, you contract the back, squeezing the muscles together and therefore strengthening them. This exercise both mimics the rowing motion and helps strengthen your back muscles in a controlled environment without any unexpected variables. For exercise instructions, please see page 138.

Reverse Ab Crunch

It is important to strengthen opposing muscle groups in order to avoid injury. Your abs are part of your core. Since we have been working the back, it is essential to spend some time on the abs. By strengthening your core muscles you will more efficiently row, engaging your entire body and strength to assist in the repetitive motion. For exercise instructions, please see page 155.

Sprint Curl

Arm strength is essential for paddling. Pulling the oars through the water in a consistent, even, and continuous motion is much more strenuous and exhausting than it sounds. Remember, this movement is propelling your boat forward through the water. It's not just strength that makes the paddling movement powerful, it is also timing and rhythm. Practicing helps to both increase arm strength and get accustomed to the timing. To train the paddling muscles we will work the biceps, the upper back, and the shoulders. Sprint curls allow you to move at a consistent, fast pace while pulling weight—similar to the motion and weight that you will experience while paddling through water. For exercise instructions, please see page 149.

Lying-Down Pull-Up, Overhand Grip

Strength in your upper arms, chest, and shoulders is essential for rowing. The pull-up requires a lot of strength (enough to pull your weight) and is great training for your upper body. For exercise instructions, please see page 139.

Standard Push-Up

Though seemingly focused on building arm strength, the push-up is a full-body exercise. You engage everything from your arms, chest, and back to your glutes and quads. It is great for strength conditioning. For exercise instructions, please see page 141.

You should perform these paddling-specific exercises at least twice a week in addition to your regular fitness routine. You only need to do 1 set of each, but you should do them all in a row with a one-minute recovery time between exercises.

Running

I consistently hear from casual runners—by casual I mean not marathon runners, but rather the woman who runs three to five miles a day to stay in shape—"I run every day, but I still have fat to lose and I can't seem to get my muscles toned." Well, you may run every day, but you aren't challenging your body by changing up your program, which keeps muscles guessing and increases calorie burn and fat loss. And you aren't lifting any weight to tone your muscles. Running is a repetitive movement. All you are doing is propelling your body forward in a motion that your body is used to, as we do the same motion at a much slower pace every day when walking.

While running is a great way to keep aerobically fit, it is notoriously hard on your bones and joints. Injury is common among runners, especially long-distance runners. In fact, long-distance runners are arguably affected by more injuries than athletes involved in any other sport—including football, volleyball, and basketball.

Running is a high-contact sport. You may not be running into other people, but you are running hard into the ground. Every time your feet hit the ground, your body is enduring an impact of three times your body weight slammed into your feet, ankles, knees, hips, and lower back. The constant pounding can create microtrauma on the shock-absorbing tissues, which over time can result in weakened tissues and cartilage, making them more prone to injury.

With resistance exercises, you can increase your running ability—your strength, endurance, energy level, muscle control, balance, and stability—while burning more calories and fat and toning your muscles.

Unlike strength training for other sports and activities, you should not do exercises that mimic the movements associated with running. Running is already working the required muscle groups; strength training those muscles can further stress the muscles and tendons, making them even more prone to injury.

Instead of focusing on the major muscle groups involved in running, you should focus on strengthening the supporting, opposing muscles.

Contrary to popular belief, strength exercises for runners are best performed in a slow and controlled manner using higher weight and lower reps and sets. Moving faster will not make you move faster when running. The purpose of strength training is to increase muscle and skeletal strength, while running is for cardio endurance. There's no need to incorporate a cardio workout into your strength practice. In fact, racing through strength exercises can actually limit the exercises' full potential. Moving slowly forces the working muscle to fully experience the movement, allowing the exercise to get into every muscle fiber. Slower movements require tension to be consistently placed on the muscle in order to complete the exercise, while fast movements can reduce muscle tension and turn the exercise into one that is less about strength and more about momentum. To ensure that you are getting the full benefit from each movement, focus on lengthening the time of each rep to six seconds—two seconds for the up motion and four seconds for the down motion. You want to exaggerate the down motion because that is the motion that is often skipped. Flexing your muscle on the up motion, then dropping it on the down is not what we want. Control the movement all the way up and all the way down to maximize the movement and the results.

Toe Raise

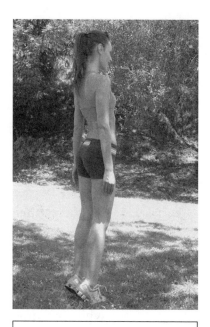

Runners tend to have very developed calf muscles and weaker shins. To avoid shin splints (small pull or tears in the shin muscle) or, even worse, a torn Achilles tendon, it is important to strengthen the shin muscles. Toe raises also help with balance.

MOVEMENT
- Stand straight with your feet hip-width apart.
- Engage your shins and raise your heels, balancing on the balls of your feet.
- Slowly and with control, lower your heels back to the starting position.
- Repeat 20 to 35 times, until your shins are exhausted.

Up the Ante

Add Weight

Holding dumbbells can quickly increase the difficulty of the squats. Start with 5-pound weights in each hand. Just be sure to maintain correct form in order to avoid injury.

Squat

Maintaining strength in both your quads and hamstrings is essential for running. Doing slow squats helps keep the movement controlled, allowing for proper strength building while minimizing your risk of a strain or tear. For exercise instructions, please see page 158.

Single-Arm Bent-Over Row

Bent-over rows focus on the middle- and upper-back muscles. Because there is no back support in the bent-over position, to minimize chances of injury, it is best to perform this exercise using one arm at a time, with the other arm on the bench to support the back. Be careful when choosing the amount of weight to lift. I prefer dumbbells to barbells because the pressure placed on your lower back when using a barbell is as much ten times the weight of the barbell. That is a lot of compression and stress and can translate to weakness and injury. Runners in particular have to be gentle with their lower back due to the stress caused by the running motion. For exercise instructions, please see page 136.

Sprint Curl

Running uses minimal arm strength. The only movement in the arms is the back-and-forth swinging motion that helps propel you forward and gives your body direction and momentum. Strengthening the arms helps to create a more balanced body and gives you more power to pull your body forward. For exercise instructions, please see page 149.

Tricep Dip

Because neither the bicep nor the tricep is focused on while running, both groups need to be exercised equally while strength training. For exercise instructions, please see page 151.

Modified Bicycle

Strengthening your oblique muscles (the muscles along the sides of your abs) will help build core strength. Your core is your powerhouse. Any exercise you do engages your core in some way, shape, or form. Running is no exception. Be sure that your core, and particularly your obliques, is strong and toned in order to minimize cramps. For exercise instructions, please see page 157.

Yoga

You may think that yoga and weight training are so completely different that the concept of their ever meeting in the middle, let alone supporting each other, is impossible. Wrong. Yoga isn't just about stretching and bending and slowly moving the body into meditative poses. It is also more than the image of the Gumby-like yogini who can easily slip her feet behind her head and is so flexible you wonder if she is actually made of rubber bands.

While there are several types of yoga, most demand strength—both physical and mental—to correctly execute the poses. Yoga is not a competitive sport, and you should not ever compare yourself to another practitioner, but the reason you might not be able to do a pose as well as your neighbor is not necessarily because you lack flexibility or balance, but because you may not have the same strength that she has. Keep in mind that balance requires a tremendous amount of strength in the small supporting muscles. Weight lifting can target the small supporting and large main muscles that can help you be a better yogini. Avoid focusing on the frustration of not being able to do the pose with correct form and you might be able to concentrate on your breathing and the calming connection between body and spirit.

To increase the benefits of the weight training, do 3 sets of 12 to 16 reps using low weight (5- to 8-pound weights are great). This way you can really hone in on a specific muscle group without bulking it. You also want to practice your yoga breathing—deep belly breaths in through your nose and long slow exhales through your nose.

Tricep Kickback

Your triceps are one of the main muscle groups engaged repeatedly during most yoga classes. They allow you to go from plank down into chaturanga and up into downward-facing dog. After several repetitions of this series, your triceps will definitely feel the burn. You can strengthen them with tricep kickbacks, making it easier for you to flow through the poses. For exercise instructions, please see page 152.

Standing Bicep Curl with Twist

Now that you have worked your triceps, you need to strengthen your biceps. The bicep curl with the added twist motion engages your bicep and the muscles between your bicep and tricep. For exercise instructions, please see page 148.

Bench Press

The shoulders are a major muscle group consistently used in yoga. If you have ever heard someone compliment a yogini for having great "yoga arms" that is because yoga creates strong pronounced shoulders that dip into thin, toned arms. The bench press can help strengthen your shoulder muscles. For exercise instructions, please see page 143.

Wall Sit with Inner-Thigh Squeeze

It is important to strengthen and stretch your inner thighs as part of your yoga conditioning. Many of the poses in a traditional yoga practice utilize your inner thighs, quads, and hamstrings. The wall sit may seem like a simple pose, but it takes intense muscle strength. For exercise instructions, please see page 170.

Tennis

Tennis is a power sport that incorporates the entire body in quick motions. You dash to one corner of the court, stop on a dime, and swing your racquet with all your might. You are using your quads, hamstrings, calves, core, biceps, and triceps in power movements that require all of your energy.

Tennis is not gentle. It is hard on your muscles, bones, and ligaments. Weight training for tennis will help strengthen the entire body, focusing on the small supporting muscles that help with those power moves. Weight training is also used to help increase power endurance—that is, your ability to continuously expel such great amounts of energy and muscular strength to power through an entire tennis match.

4-Count Jump Squat

Jump squats help strengthen the quads, glutes, and hamstrings, mimicking the motion tennis players engage in while standing ready to hit the ball. For exercise instructions, please see page 177.

4-Count Jump Lunge

Jump lunges strengthen the quads and hamstrings, mimicking a quick sprint across the tennis court. For exercise instructions, please see page 174.

Standard Push-Up

Push-ups focus on the chest, but they also target the shoulders, arms, back, and glutes. They help train your upper body to power through each strike of the ball. For exercise instructions, please see page 141.

Sprint Curl

The arm motion in tennis is quick and powerful, jolting the muscles, bones, and ligaments. Sprint curls teach you to quickly move weight in a controlled and exact manner. For exercise instructions, please see page 149.

Now use your new resistance-built strength to get out there and get your game on!

Index